# THE FITNESS FORMULA

## By Steve Sokol ... The World's Fittest Man

The Secret to Health, Fitness, and Success
Through Proper Nutrition and Exercise
for the World's Active and Busy Families

**Sponsored by:**

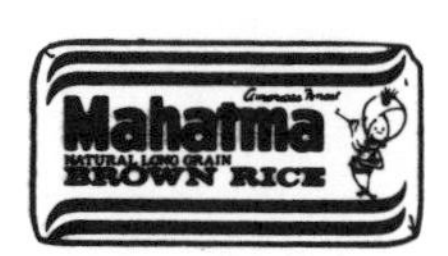


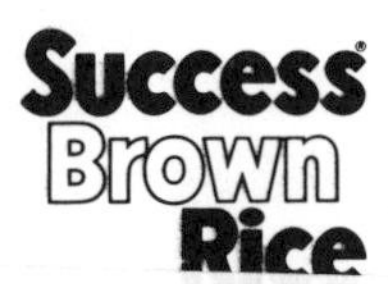

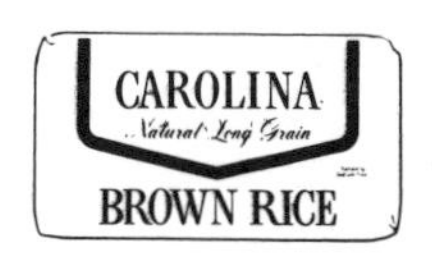


A GLOBAL HEALTH PUBLICATION

**The Fitness Formula**

This information is not presented with the intention of diagnosing or prescribing. It is intended to help one cooperate with his physician in a mutual desire to build and maintain health. In the event one uses this information without his doctor's approval, he is prescribing for himself. This is his constitutional right, but the author, publisher, and distributors assume no responsibility.



Global Health Ltd.
Box 18, Site 1, R.R. 2
Tofield, Alberta, Canada
T0B 4J0

Canadian Cataloguing in Publication Data
Sokol, Steven David, 1956
The Fitness Formula
Includes Index
ISBN 0-921202-06-7
1. Nutrition. Dietary supplements. 2. Exercise
I. Global Health Ltd. II. Title
RA784 613.7 C90-091315-0

Printed in the United States of America

# Table of Contents

# Dedication

I dedicate this book to my parents, Simon and Bernice, who have been behind me every step of the way and taught me to aspire toward my dreams. And to my brothers Lanny and Barry and my wife Leslie, who are there to remind me what hard work is all about and motivate me through the rough times. I love these people more than words can describe.

Steve Sokol

# Introduction

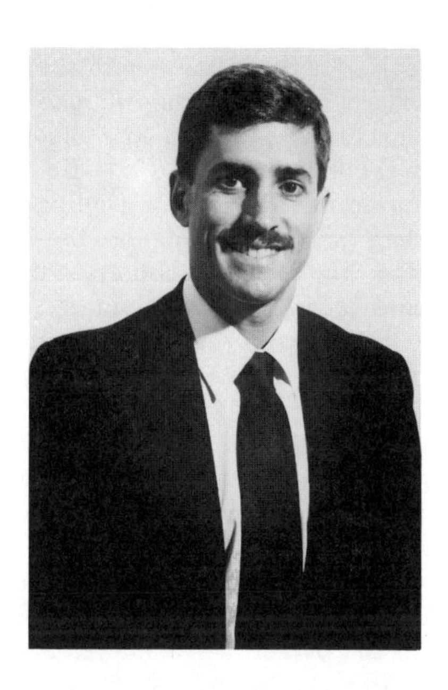

**About The Author: The World's Fittest Man**

At the age of eight, sickly Steve Sokol began a daily swimming workout at his doctor's request: it was a last-ditch attempt to relieve some of the symptoms of severe childhood asthma. Fifteen short years later he did more than 52,000 consecutive sit-ups in just over thirty-two hours.

Today, he holds more than twenty official world fitness records — and has been dubbed "the world's fittest man." And, needless to say, there's no trace of asthma.

A miracle?

Maybe. But it's a "miracle" that was forged with plenty of sheer determination — along with pounding perseverance, incredible nutritional know-how, a huge dose of willpower, and the academic training to make it all work.

The "sickly little kid" that the doctor sent to the swimming pool kept on swimming. In fact, he swam competitively on a varsity level throughout high school and college. That college was Tufts University, where he earned an honors degree in chemical engineering. From there he pursued a career in engineering with International Business Machines. And, of course, he kept on exercising.

The turning point for Sokol came with the chance to do a charity stunt at a local mall. Sokol signed up to take pledges for all the sit-ups he could do at a San Jose shopping mall, with proceeds going to the American Red Cross. He prepared for the event by chalking up more than half a million sit-ups in the fifteen weeks before the event. Going into the Red Cross fund-raiser he predicted that he would obliterate the then-current world sit-up record set in 1976 by "Captain America" Jones: 51,001 sit-ups in three days, a rate of 650 sit-ups per hour. His goal, he stated, was "to be the best at something."

If nobody took Sokol seriously as the Red Cross fund-raiser began, they soon changed their minds. Twenty-four-year-old Sokol was doing bent-knee sit-ups with a vengeance. Crowds of shoppers who stopped to watch wondered how long he could possibly keep up the pace.

As he passed the twenty-four-hour mark and the 45,000 repetition mark, the tears started. The pain, as one reporter put it, had "exceeded the bounds of human endurance." Despite being slathered with Vaseline and baby oil, the skin on his back blistered and cracked; his backside was rubbed raw. His composure was demolished.

In an account given to *Nautilus Magazine,* Sokol recounted that "I thought I was losing it. I was getting out of control."

But did he stop?

No ... not even close. He went on to establish what *Nautilus* termed "a new pinnacle for abdominal abuse." In front of fitness officials and swarms of curious onlookers, Sokol finished 52,003 bent-leg sit-ups in thirty-two hours, seventeen minutes. In a word, he left Captain America in the dust — Sokol averaged 1,600 sit-ups per hour.

The victory didn't come cheap. Sokol was feverish for three days. It was a full week before he could sit in a chair. And it was six weeks before he fully recovered from the stunt.

But, he told a *Wall Street Journal* reporter, after the event "Something just clicked in my head. I didn't like what I was doing as an engineer. I thought I could formulate a career for myself as an athlete."

Sokol put his mind — and his incredibly fit body — to the task, and started working toward his goal of becoming a fitness expert. A mere four months after the Red Cross fund-raiser, he set another record: this time he did 13,013 consecutive leg-lifts in five hours and forty-five minutes for the Westchester (New York) Division of the American Cancer Society.

As the *Wall Street Journal* tells it, for the next two years Sokol "sweated his way into the public eye," occasionally receiving free health-club memberships, vitamins, and running shoes. There were more records in those two years, too: 30,000 jumping jacks in seven and a half hours, 3,333 squat thrusts in four hours, and 1,001 sit-ups in thirty-nine minutes — with a forty-two-pound weight on his chest.

Not surprisingly, Sokol began to attract nationwide publicity. In December 1983 he provided the sweat and tears while the community of San Jose provided the blood: Sokol set a new world record by riding a stationary bicycle 500.2 miles in less than twenty-four hours for a Red Cross blood drive. Sokol pedaled away at a local radio station to publicize the need for blood during the holidays — and to encourage San Jose residents to donate blood at El Paseo Shopping Center.

As he climbed off the bicycle at the end of the event, he quipped, "I really felt like quitting several times. This was almost as hard as the sit-up record."

But Sokol's not a quitter — and he seems to have a flair for executing events that are bigger and better than the previous ones he conquers. If he could pedal 500.2 miles on a stationary bicycle, he reasoned, why not on a regulation bike? And, since he was committed to charity, why not for a charity close to his heart — asthma? Just six months after conquering the stationary bicycle, Sokol pedaled the 500.2 miles from San Francisco to Los Angeles in forty-three hours and eight minutes. A crew of five followed in a motor home, handing him food and drink; Sokol ate with one hand and steered with the other. And he did it all for pledges to Camp Superstuff, a camp for asthmatic kids.

But that's not all: he completed the entire ride *without once sitting down on the bicycle seat.*

Sokol's dream was becoming reality: he worked toward a master's degree in advanced exercise physiology at San Jose State University. He worked out six days a week, four to six hours a day. He began promoting exercise gear. And he began earning his living as an athlete and fitness consultant. And, of course, he kept setting records.

For one, he completed an "electronic triathlon" — going the same distances as those in the Hawaii World Ironman Championship on a treadmill (26.2 miles), a stationary bicycle (112 miles), and a rowing machine (4 miles). He ran, cycled, and rowed a total of 142.2 miles in eight hours, fifty-seven minutes, and two seconds, establishing the standard for an electronic triathlon. (He had previously completed Hawaii's Ironman Triathlon twice — once in twelve hours.)

As the years came, so did the records. He bettered his own time in sit-ups, leg-lifts, squat thrusts, and jumping jacks. He did 3,170 sit-ups in one hour in front of 250 astonished onlookers at a sporting goods show at the New York Coliseum. He worked for five and a half continuous hours on a Nordic Track ski simulator. He climbed 40,000 vertical feet on a versa climber in just under five hours — and later climbed 13,120 vertical feet at the New Orleans Hilton in one hour.

Sokol's goal is to educate people about fitness — and to serve as a role model for people struggling to achieve physical fitness. Does he expect others to do what he does? Absolutely not, he says. "But if someone sees me do 3,100 sit-ups in an hour, it might inspire him to do 50 sit-ups each morning."

Sokol has been featured on news programs throughout the nation, and has appeared on "Sports Talk," "Claim to Fame," "AM San Francisco," and "The Late Show with Joan Rivers," among others. He was one of eight athletes worldwide selected to compete on NBC's "Survival of the Fittest."

Stories about Sokol have appeared in *Sports Illustrated*, *The Wall Street Journal*, *Sport Magazine*, *Advertising Age*, *Sports Fitness*, *Cosmopolitan*, *The New York Times*, *The New York Post*, *The Chicago Sun Times*, *The Denver Post*, and *The Dallas Morning News*. He is a talented writer and speaker, and conducts seminars for audiences across the nation on the topics of health, nutrition, weight training, flexibility, stress reduction, and a variety of sports.

In addition to holding more than twenty fitness records, Sokol is an avid competitor in endurance events. He twice completed the Hawaii Ironman Triathlon, with a best time of twelve hours.

He finished the 1980 Pepsi of Reno-Lake Tahoe seventy-two-mile run in fifteen hours, forty-five minutes. And he finished seventh place in the 1981 L.A. Wheelmen Triple Century Bicycle Race, clocking three hundred miles in twenty-three and a half hours.

As the *Wall Street Journal* so aptly stated, "all this toil hasn't gone unnoticed." In addition to being dubbed "The World's Fittest Man," Sokol was named by *Nautilus Magazine* as having "the world's most durable stomach," and *Cosmopolitan* once selected him as "Bachelor of the Month."

In addition to setting records, working out six hours a day, studying, writing, and making numerous promotional appearances, Sokol is busy with — and most proud of — his work with charities. He is a national spokesman for the Arthritis Foundation, works regionally with the American Lung Association, and has worked extensively with the American Red Cross, the American Heart Association, the American Cancer Society, and several smaller foundations. Sokol has also combined efforts with the Sports Club in working with the National Fitness Foundation and Athletes For Kids. Steve is presently the fitness director and education specialist for two West Coast fitness clubs.

Here, Sokol shares with you the basics of general nutrition and health; the special nutritional needs of athletes; and down-to-earth information for people of all skill levels who want to get fit by improving strength, endurance, flexibility, and cardiovascular fitness.

# You Are What You Eat: General Nutrition Guidelines

Remember the old saying, "You are what you eat"?

Maybe you've never paid much attention — or taken it too seriously.

If so, it's time to change your way of thinking!

The food you eat — the nutrition that fuels your body — determines to a very real extent not only how you look, but how you feel, how well your body can work for you, and even how susceptible you are to illness.

Nutrition is a key factor in what I like to call a "health and fitness lifestyle." *Health* and *fitness* are not the same thing; I like to think of them as separate pieces in an overall puzzle.

Health is defined by Webster's Dictionary as "the absence of disease and pain." Fitness, from an exercise physiologist's point of view, is combination of aerobic endurance, muscular strength and endurance, and joint flexibility. Obviously, they're not the same — and you can have one without the other.

How?

Consider a high school wrestler who is forced to drop a quick twenty pounds before a championship meet. He's undoubtedly very fit — he's got great muscle strength and outstanding joint flexibility. But he's also probably unhealthy: his drastic weight-loss efforts have left him malnourished and dehydrated.

Or look at the sedentary, slightly overweight, middle-aged office manager. He's probably healthy; the doctor gave him a clean bill of health at his annual checkup. But he would undoubtedly score very poorly on a basic fitness test.

To be at your best, you need both health *and* fitness. And you need to live a health and fitness lifestyle.

Sound complicated?

It isn't. In fact, its simplicity is beautiful. It can be summed up in a few short sentences: Eat a nutritious, well-balanced diet. Get regular exercise. Reduce the amount of stress in your life. Get adequate rest. And eliminate (or drastically reduce) the harmful elements in your life — alcohol, drug abuse, cigarette smoking, chewing tobacco, and so on.

Come on, you might say — *nobody* is perfect. You're right! I'm not asking you to be perfect. The idea is to optimize wherever you can so that you compensate for the indulgences. The net result should be a comfortable pattern of living that helps you be at your best.

Here's how it works: Maybe you crave sweets. Maybe you aren't willing to completely eliminate them from your diet. You might be willing to compensate by cutting back and by taking some other healthful steps — reducing extra fat (such as butter or red meat), exercising more to burn the extra calories, or cutting out the beer you used to have with dinner.

The important thing to remember is that a "health and fitness lifestyle" is not a two-week program. It's not a two-month program. It's a permanent change in the way you live — a change that will bring tremendous benefits in the way you feel and perform.

This book will give you the suggestions you need to get you started. To begin, let's take a look at two of the basics: nutrition and exercise.

## Exploding the Calorie Myth

If you're old enough to count, you know about calories. We as Americans are a calorie-conscious society. It's estimated that more than 50 million American men and 60 million American women are overweight. More than half of us are trying to lose weight at any given time. And there are more than 17,000 fad diets on the market — many of them based on extreme calorie restriction.

Unfortunately, there are some widely believed myths about calories — and until you understand the facts, you won't be able to count calories to your advantage.

First, exactly what is a *calorie*?

One k-cal (food calorie) is the amount of energy needed to raise the temperature of one kilogram of water one degree centigrade. The energy that food provides, then, is measured in calories. A small apple measures in at 40 calories; a small wedge of cheesecake nets 400.

Weight loss and weight gain is based on a simple, unchangeable law: if you consume more calories than your body needs for its energy demands, your body will store the extra as fat. It takes about 15 kcals per pound per day to maintain a given body weight.

It sounds pretty simple, then: if you want to lose weight, cut back on calories, right?

Right — to a degree. And that's where the popular myths about calories come into the picture.

The first myth says that if you want to lose weight in a hurry, just do a drastic cut in the amount of calories you consume every day. According to the myth (and tens of thousands of fad diets that hold it sacred), the fewer calories you eat, the faster you'll lose weight.

It simply doesn't work that way. Why? Blame your metabolism. Your metabolism contains some kind of inborn mechanism that knows how much fuel your body needs to function at its prime. As long as it gets what it needs, it's happy. But when it is suddenly deprived — when you drastically cut back on the amount of calories you consume — your metabolism kicks into a "survival" mode. In other words, it does what it determines necessary to protect you against starvation.

Here's what happens: It puts your appetite into overdrive so you'll eat more; as a result, you feel ravenously hungry. (Ever wonder why you get so hungry when you start to "diet"?) It stubbornly holds on to its fat stores; instead, it gives up muscle tissue, body fluid, and , in extremes, tissue from your organs. It makes you slow down and conserve energy so you won't burn off any calories, as a result, you feel tired. And, finally, your metabolism itself slows down to preciously save whatever you do toss in its direction; as a result, you lose very little weight.

The final analysis? The fewer calories you eat, the more your body struggles to keep you from losing weight.

So how is weight loss possible? You need to fuel your body adequately in order for your metabolism to speed up. Try eating three to six small meals a day instead of one large one; having food in your system will keep your metabolism stimulated and will keep your rate of calorie burn high. Having food in your system on a regular basis also gives your metabolism less of a need to store food as fat. Your metabolism no longer believes you're starving, so it no longer acts to "protect" you.

A moderately active 150-pound thirty-year-old needs about

2,200 calories a day to maintain that weight. He needs more if he gets regular vigorous exercise or is extremely active. You should determine what your daily calorie needs are and you should eat a variety of wholesome foods to meet that need. If you need to lose weight, you should aim for a loss of no more than one to two pounds per week. *You should never eat fewer than 1,200 calories per day unless under strict medical observation.*

That leads to the other popular myth about calories: whether it comes from broccoli or pizza, a calorie is a calorie.

Wrong. All calories are *not* created equal. Calories that come from fat sources (like butter, cheese, and red meat) make you fatter than calories that come from complex carbohydrates (like broccoli) or lean proteins (like chicken). Your body has a greater tendency to store "fat" calories as body fat than the calories you get from fruits, vegetables, grains, and other sources.

Let's put it this way: if you're aiming for 1,200 calories a day, you could eat a chocolate milkshake, a piece of cherry cheese-cake, and a small slice of chocolate cake. That would do it. Or you could eat three well-balanced meals and a few low-fat snacks. Both ways, you'd get 1,200 calories. But you wouldn't lose weight both ways.

**The Bathroom Scale: Only Part of the Story**

Weight gain does not always signal a gain in body fat.

Why?

There are some fairly obvious examples. A weight-lifter and a pregnant woman will both show an increase on the bathroom scale, but no increase in body fat — the weight-lifter is experiencing an increase in muscle mass, and the pregnant woman is tipping the scales due to a developing baby.

More important than how much you weigh is how much body fat is stored in your tissues. The amount of fat in the tissues is expressed as a "percentage" of body fat — in other words, what percentage of your body is fatty tissue. The average body fat levels of healthy men and women are 12 to 15 percent for men and 18 to 22 percent for women. Athletes, who tend to be lean and muscular, may have 10 percent or less body fat for men and 10 to 14 percent for women.

Your physician can help you determine your body fat percentage. A man should not be below 3 percent or over 22 percent; a woman should not be below 10 percent or over 28 percent. Levels that exceed these extremes are considered unhealthy.

### Nutritional Guidelines for a Well-Balanced Diet

According to estimates, one in every five men and one in every three women in this country are obese — they exceed their desirable weight by more than 20 percent. A big culprit, say the experts, is diet. Most Americans get 40 percent of their daily calories from fat—two to three times the recommended percentage. And instead of getting 70 percent from carbohydrates, they get a paltry 40 percent — and half of that is refined sugar.

Obesity is only one result of the average American diet. The others read like a shopping list of today's leading killers: coronary heart disease, stroke, diabetes, high blood pressure, and cancer. With proper diet, these killers can be at least partially — if not completely — prevented.

What constitutes a "proper" diet?

Nutritional experts have set up general guidelines that give a recommended balance of nutrients. According to those guidelines, you should get 15 to 20 percent of your daily calories from fat; 60 to 70 percent from carbohydrates; and 15 to 20 percent from lean protein. You should get no more than 300 mg cholesterol per day (most Americans get two to three times that much).

### Fats

Fats do not contain nutrients; they simply contain calories. Most Americans eat far too many fats in their diets —you should aim for no more than 15 to 20 percent of your calories coming from fats each day.

If fats are so bad, why not cut them completely from your diet?

Fat *does* have a function in the body in moderate amounts. It insulates you from the cold; it cushions and protects your vital organs; it provides energy; and it carries the fat-soluble vitamins. But when your diet is too high in fats, the problems begin.

There are two basic kinds of fats in the diet: saturated fats and unsaturated fats.

**Saturated Fats.** Saturated fats (which includes cholesterol) are those fats that are solid at room temperature. Sources of saturated fats include red meat, the skin of poultry, eggs, shellfish, margarine, and whole dairy products (such as butter, cream, cheese, and milk). Saturated fats also include hydrogenated vegetable oils, such as vegetable oil shortening. Cholesterol and other saturated fats cause the buildup of plaque deposits in the arteries, leading to atherosclerosis.

Cholesterol is a waxy yellowish substance composed of fats and a certain kind of protein (known as lipoproteins). Essential to human life, it is manufactured by the body and found in every cell in the body. Cholesterol gives rigidity to the cell walls and is essential in producing hormones. Your body manufactures as much cholesterol as it needs — so when your diet is high in cholesterol, it's no longer needed in the cells. Instead, it's deposited in the bloodstream, where is can eventually choke the arteries and starve your vital organs of needed oxygen.

There are two basic kinds of lipoproteins in cholesterol. Low-density lipoproteins (LDLs) are the culprits that cause heart disease; high-density lipoproteins (HDLs) are the "good guys" that promote the removal of cholesterol from the body.

If you haven't had a blood test to determine your cholesterol levels, do it today! Ideally, your cholesterol level should be around 150; anything under 200 is acceptable, but scientists have found that at levels under 150, plaque deposits may actually reverse. You should try to keep your LDL to HDL ratio less than 2 to 1, and your triglycerides should be below 100. You can reduce your cholesterol levels significantly by making changes in your diet and exercise habits; your physician can prescribe medication if your cholesterol level is extremely high. It's worth it to bring the level down: for every 1 percent drop in cholesterol levels, you reduce your risk of heart disease by 2 percent.

**Unsaturated Fats.** Unsaturated fats (polyunsaturated and monounsaturated fats) come from plant sources and are liquid at room temperature; they include olive oil, peanut oil, soybean oil, corn oil, fish oils, and other liquid vegetable oils. Safflower oil is one of the best. Unsaturated fats don't boost your cholesterol levels, but they are high in calories without providing nutrients. Eat too much unsaturated fat, and you'll gain weight — plus you'll have a difficult time losing it later.

What should your target fat consumption be?

As stated earlier, you should get no more than 15 to 20 percent of your daily calories in the form of fat. Let's put that into perspective: 75 percent of the calories in red meat are saturated fats. From 50 to 75 percent of the calories in cheese are saturated fats. Ideally, your diet should contain equal parts of saturated fats (those in meat, cheese and dairy products), monounsaturated fats (such as olive and peanut oil), and polyunsaturated fats (such as fish oils and liquid vegetable oils). Try for the equivalent of about a tablespoon of each per day.

If you're an average American, you should try to cut your total fat intake in half — and your total cholesterol intake by three-fourths.

How?

Cut down on the amount of red meat you eat; substitute fish and poultry that has had the skin removed. Drink skim milk; stick to nonfat yogurt and low-fat or non-fat cottage cheese. Avoid using butter or stick margarine — try margarine in a squeeze bottle. Reduce or eliminate egg yolks and cheeses. Stay away from shortening, palm oil, and coconut oil — all three cause your body to produce more cholesterol.

### Carbohydrates

The bulk of your diet — 60 percent for most people, and up to 70 percent for athletes — should come from carbohydrates, which serve as your main source of fuel. Carbohydrates help maintain the protein in your tissues, and your central nervous system functions almost exclusively on carbohydrates.

There are basically two kinds of carbohydrates: complex carbohydrates and refined or simple carbohydrates.

**Complex Carbohydrates.** Complex carbohydrates come from unprocessed fruits, vegetables, and grains (including rice, breads, pastas, and cereals). They are almost ideal as foods: they are low in fat, contain no sodium, are rich in vitamins, and are an excellent source of fiber. Simply stated they fill you up without filling you out.

There's another advantage to complex carbohydrates: they are broken down into simple sugars in the body, but the breakdown is gradual. Your body gets a steady, regulated source of fuel instead of the erratic "sugar rush" that happens when you munch on a candy bar.

But that's not all — as mentioned, complex carbohydrates are an excellent source of dietary fiber. What does that mean to you? The bulk from the fiber helps you feel full and satisfied longer; you won't be as prone to overeat. It also aids in digestion and elimination. And the soluble fiber from fruits, vegetables, and whole grains helps lower your cholesterol levels. Oat bran, wheat bran, rice bran and the pectin in fruits are especially beneficial.

You need two to four grams of fiber a day for optimum health. To give you an idea, one cup of All Bran cereal provides two grams of fiber; so do three carrots or three apples.

**Refined Carbohydrates.** You know these as sugars — candy bars, cakes, cookies, pies, and so on. No more than 10 percent of your carbohydrate allowance should come from this group. Why? For lots of reasons. First, refined carbohydrates are "empty calories" — they provide plenty of calories, but no nutrition. They cause tooth decay. And they cause a rapid rise in blood sugar that is followed by a surge of insulin from the pancreas and an ensuing drop in blood sugar. The result? You eat a candy bar, with 200 to 300 calories, but you're satisfied only briefly. A few minutes later, you're hungry again.

Refined carbohydrates in low concentrations can be used to provide energy during endurance exercise. *Beware* — These refined carbohydrates often contain much fat as well as sugar — A double whammy! Pastries, cookies, and cakes all have a lot of fat.

I like to think of complex carbohydrates as almost-perfect foods — but I have to add the reminder that it's possible to spoil almost-perfect foods. Take the humble potato as an example. One medium baked potato provides about 70 calories — all of them stemming from complex carbohydrates. What happens if you cut that medium potato into French fries and deep fry them? The humble potato now weighs in at 240 calories — two-thirds of them from fat. Wait — there's more. What if you slice that medium potato into thin potato chips and fry those? You're now up to a whopping 440 calories — 85 percent of them from fat.

The same is true of rice — if we fry it in oil and add pork and eggs it is a high fat food, but if boiled it is virtually fat free and very high in complex carbohydrates.

## Protein

Ideally, you should get the same percentage of calories from protein as you do from fats — 15 to 20 percent of your daily calories is considered optimal. Proteins are generally found in both animal and vegetable foods, although plant proteins are usually "incomplete" and need to be eaten in combination.

No one can argue that protein is an essential nutrient. Protein contains amino acids, which are the basic building blocks of the body. Amino acids enable the production of hormones and enzymes; they maintain, repair, and grow tissues. Protein itself makes up the cell nucleus and the membranes, including those of the skin, tendons, ligaments, and muscles. Of the twenty-two amino acids needed by the body, nine are considered "essential" — in other words, the body can't manufacture them. They must be obtained through the diet.

If protein is so great, why should it be so limited in the diet?

Good question — and there's an equally good answer. Simply stated, too much of it is harmful. Protein breaks down into urea and uric acid, highly toxic substances that must be eliminated from the body by the kidneys; if you eat too much protein, you run a very real risk of kidney damage. An excess of protein is converted to fat and stored in the cells.

That's not all. Protein, once touted by athletes as the perfect pre-competition food, is actually a very poor source of energy. And, unfortunately, many conventional sources of protein — such as red meat and eggs — are also foods that are high in fats.

Generally, the recommended daily allowance of protein is .8 grams per kilogram of body weight. Since a kilogram is roughly equal to 2.2 pounds, a 152-pound man would need 56 grams of protein per day; a 112-pound woman would need 40 grams per day. Use 1 gram of protein per kilogram to be insured adequate protein.

While most athletes do not require more protein, new research shows that endurance athletes should beef up their protein allowance to between 1.5 and 2.0 grams per kilogram of body weight. Bodybuilders and other strength athletes may also benefit from this extra protein allotment.

### Vitamins and Minerals

Vitamins and minerals — which are present in rich supply in a nutritious, well-balanced diet — do not supply energy to your body, but are necessary for energy metabolism. Minerals also help regulate the chemical reactions in the cells, and are critical to the muscles' ability to relax and contract.

Do you need to take a vitamin/mineral supplement?

I use supplements regularly, and I recommend a complete multi-vitamin/multi-mineral supplement. You need to remember, however, that *nutritional supplements do not take the place of food.* Nutritional supplements, in fact, are only catalysts — they need to work along with food in order to be effective. Always take a nutritional supplement with a meal.

I like to think of nutritional supplements as an "insurance policy" against inadequate nutrition. In simple terms, I eat a well-balanced diet from all four food groups, and use my nutritional supplement as insurance, or added protection.

There are some important guidelines to consider when using nutritional supplements. First, remember that too much of anything is unhealthy. Avoid megadoses of vitamins and minerals. Your supplement should provide no more than 100 percent of the recommended daily allowance of key nutrients. The fat-soluble vitamins — A, D, E, and K — and many minerals are toxic if taken in high doses.

Second, some people in certain situations have an increased need for extra vitamins. Vegetarians should increase their dose of vitamin $B_{12}$ in order to prevent pernicious anemia. Take extra vitamin C if you are recovering from an injury or illness. You should also take extra B-complex and vitamin C if you are under stress (either emotional or physical), since these are water-soluble vitamins and are excreted more rapidly through perspiration and urine when the body is under stress.

If you are extremely active, boost your dosage of vitamin C on the days that you work out or exercise. You should aim for 1 gram of vitamin C for each hour that you exercise.

Finally, there are some circumstances under which minerals should be increased. Women need extra calcium to help prevent osteoporosis (a loss of calcium from the bone); 1000 mg per day is a baseline dosage. Women, as well as competitive runners, also need extra iron to prevent anemia; always take iron with vitamin C to aid in absorption. If you are physically active, you also need extra potassium to prevent muscle cramping; bananas and oranges are excellent sources of natural potassium.

*Never take salt or sodium supplements.* You'll get plenty of sodium on the foods you eat, even if you never use a salt shaker. Too much sodium causes blood pressure to skyrocket and can cause water retention.

**Water**

One of the most important foods you can include in your diet is pure, simple water. Approximately 60 percent of your body is composed of water, and it's needed for all body functions. Water is especially critical for preventing dehydration during exercise.

There are other important reasons why you need lots of water. If your diet is rich in carbohydrates, as it should be, you need extra water. Why? Carbohydrates that are stored in the muscles need to bind to three times their weight in water in order to be used by the body. And a diet rich in fiber — as yours shouldbe — needs to be supplemented with plenty of water to prevent constipation.

Aim for at least eight to ten eight-ounce glasses of water a day. On days when you work out or exercise, increase that amount substantially, especially during hot weather.

**General Dietary Guidelines**

To achieve the greatest level of health and fitness, eat at least three meals each day; eating three to six small meals during the day provides you with constant energy and a level amount of blood sugar. As discussed, when you eat only one large meal during the day, your body learns to store more of your food as fat to protect you against possible starvation.

Eat most of your calories early in the day so you'll have plenty of energy for an active lifestyle. Eat fewer calories at night — your body is at rest, and will store any excess as fat.

If you need to lose weight, remember that diet alone won't do the trick — you need to combine a high-carbohydrate diet of at least 1,200 calories a day with an increase in physical exercise. If you want to gain muscle mass, add approximately 500 calories a day to your diet and lift weights for strength. (I'll discuss strength training in more detail later.)

In addition to these general guidelines, the American Cancer Society has established a set of dietary guidelines that can help protect against cancer:

1. Eat foods that are high in fiber.
2. Eat more natural sources of vitamins A and C, such as fresh vegetables and fruits.
3. Reduce your intake of fat.
4. Avoid obesity.

5. Restrict your intake of salty foods, salt-cured foods, smoked foods, and nitrate-cured foods.

**Specific Foods for Health and Fitness**

Ready for some specifics?

When you begin to eat for a health and fitness lifestyle, you'll find your options are almost endless; learn to look at the great array of delicious, healthy foods instead of concentrating on the restrictions!

For carbohydrates and fiber, which should comprise the bulk of your diet (60 to 70 percent of your daily calories), choose the following:

**Fruits and Vegetables.** Enjoy all the fruits and vegetables you want except avocados and olives, which are high in fat. Fresh fruits and veggies make great snacks — they're high in fiber, low in fat, and provide plenty of sustained energy.

For the greatest health benefits, scrub fruits and vegetables well and eat them with their skins and peels.

**Cereals.** Hot cereals — such as oatmeal, farina, and buckwheat — are rich in carbohydrates and fiber. Also choose non-sugared whole-grain cold cereals, such as Grapenuts, Shredded Wheat, Nutrigrain, and Health Valley. Try rice — hot or cold — instead of cereal now and then.

**Breads.** Heavy, coarse-grain, and whole-grain breads are best. Avoid breads that contain animal shortening; read labels, and choose breads that contain soy or safflower oil. Don't use butter or margarine on your bread.

**Pasta.** Pasta is a filling, low-fat source of energy and can be served with a variety of low-fat sauces (avoid sauces that contain butter or cream). Steer clear of egg pasta — it's too high in fat.

**Rice, potatoes, and grains.** See the rice recipes for more great ideas on page 32. Enjoy these freely. Just remember to bake, boil, or mash — don't fry!

**Beans and lentils.** Besides being a great source of carbohydrates, beans and lentils also provide protein.

For protein, which should constitute 15 to 20 percent of your daily calories, avoid proteins with excessive fat — try to limit your use of red meats, organ meats, butter, margarine, cream, egg yolks, hard cheese, all hydrogenated oils (such as shortening), fried foods, nuts, seed and mayonnaise.

Instead, choose from the following:

**Poultry.** Eat the white meat of turkey and chicken. Make sure to remove the skin first, and broil — don't fry!

**Fish.** Broiled fish is an excellent low-fat source of protein; in general, fish that swim are lower cholesterol than shellfish. Another good source is tuna packed in water. Fatty fish like salmon, tuna, and mackerel have been shown to help reduce cholesterol levels and should be included in your diet.

**Low-fat dairy products.** Choose skim milk, low-fat or non-fat cottage cheese, and nonfat yogurt.

**Eggs.** The high-fat part of the egg (and the part that contains the cholesterol) is the yolk. When you use eggs in cooking, separate them — and use the whites only.

## Exercise

Good nutrition is only part of the health and fitness lifestyle.

What's the other part?

Exercise!

Oh, great. When you're already being pulled in all directions by demands on the job and at home, how on earth can you find time to exercise?

For too many, that time never comes. It's a trap that's easy to get caught in: you feel worn out after meetings, appointments, a hectic commute, family time, and all the other "chores" that fill your day. Exercise seems like the one thing that can be moved to the back burner and dealt with later.

Don't let yourself fall into that trap! I'm not expecting you to work out for hours a day; that's a rigorous schedule that only professional athletes need to adhere to. I'm hoping to help you understand that exercise — even a moderate amount of exercise three or four times a week — packs plenty of benefits that you *need* in your life.

What kind of benefits?

There are many. For one thing, you'll look better. Your muscles will be toned, your body trim and taut, your complexion glowing. You'll have an inner vitality and zest for life that will accompany your good health. Exercise is essential to weight loss and a healthy heart and lungs. The latest research states that it well even help to lengthen your life!

Did you know that exercise is one of the best stress-busters around? It's true! Scientific research has proven that exercise negates the physical effects of stress. You'll feel better and more relaxed if you exercise regularly — and you'll have the energy and health to meet the demands you're faced with every day.

One final note: the body, literally, is "the temple of the spirit." When your body is fit and healthy, you'll do better in all aspects of your life—including thought processes and creative endeavors.

Okay, you need to exercise. How should you go about it?

*Slowly,* especially if you haven't exercised for a long time. To avoid injury and sore muscles, add no more than 5 to 10 percent per week to your total exercise program.

I'll discuss the specifics of exercise programs later, but your total conditioning program should include three basic kinds of exercise: cardiovascular exercise, to improve the health of your heart, lungs, and circulation; muscular strength and endurance exercise; and flexibility training to keep you limber and injury-free. Combining all three kinds of exercise into your workout gives you a complete total body workout.

The foundation of any exercise program should be cardiovascular — sometimes called "aerobic" — exercise. Why? It's the exercise that promotes health and long life, burns calories and fat most efficiently, reduces stress, and increases energy. Good cardiovascular exercises include fast-paced walking, jogging, cycling, swimming, rowing, and aerobics. To get the greatest benefit from cardiovascular exercise, you need to maintain you "target heart rate zone" for at least twenty continuous minutes.

To calculate your "target zone," subtract your age from 220; your target zone is 65 to 80 percent of the result. As an example, a 20-year-old would subtract 20 from 220, for a total of 200. The "target zone" would 65 to 80 percent of 200, or 130 to 160 beats per minute. A 20-year-old, then, should maintain a pulse rate of 130 to 160 for at least 20 continuous minutes for an effective aerobic workout.

To get started, set aside at least twenty minutes — more, if you can — three or four times a week. Sound impossible? It's not! Try getting up half an hour earlier in the morning, or go for a brisk walk during your lunch hour. An evening jog might fit your schedule. Or you might even hop on a stationary bike or a Nordic Track ski machine during your favorite television program.

Before and after your aerobic exercise, spend at least five

minutes stretching your muscles, especially the ones you use exercising. (If you jog, stretch your calves, the front and back of the thigh, and your lower back. If you swim, stretch your shoulders, arms, chest, and back.) Remember: stretch, *don't bounce!* Hold this stretch for thirty to sixty seconds; you should feel a good stretch, but you shouldn't feel any pain. If you do, you're stretching too far.

Stretching before you exercise warms up the muscles, prevents cramps and muscle pulls, and prepares your body for exercise. Stretching after you exercise is a good way to cool down, and prevents your muscles from tightening and cramping.

Strengthening exercises should be done three or four times a week, too — more often if you have problem areas. Since most aerobic exercises work the lower extremities, look for strengthening ("calisthenic") exercises that work the abdomen and upper body. I would suggest bent-knee sit-ups, partial sit-ups, and leg raises for the abdomen; pushups, pullups, and bar dips for the upper body; and weight exercises (such as bench press and bicep curls) for individual areas.

With half an hour a day, you can do both cardiovascular and strengthening exercises — and in that brief time, you'll reap tremendous rewards!

**Family Fitness**

Guess what? The family that plays together stays together — and exercise is a great way to improve on quality time while setting a tremendous example that can lead to life-long fitness and health.

If you want your kids to exercise regularly and stay fit, you need to show them how. It's easy! Choose activities that you enjoy; workouts should be fun, something the whole family looks forward to.

If you want to start a family fitness program, introduce your children to a broad spectrum of activities. Concentrate on "lifetime activities that the whole family can enjoy — I'd recommend walking, hiking, jogging, bicycle riding, swimming, or another activity that suits your family size, style, and preferences. Don't force your children into activities that are your favorites; encourage them to choose the things they like to do.

Your children might also enjoy individual sports, such as golf, tennis, bowling, archery, racquetball, skiing, skating, or rowing. Your choices will, of course, depend on how much you can afford to spend, what equipment is available, whether lessons can be arranged, and the climate in your area.

Don't overlook team sports: they can offer great aerobic benefits while teaching children how to work together with teammates *if* they are fun, supervised, played in a safe environment, and free of pressure. I recommend basketball, soccer, field hockey, or ice hockey. Baseball offers limited exercise value, and full contact football should not be played by young children who are still growing.

Remember that most children exercise at a level close to their maximum capacity, so your children may fatigue quickly. Children are also more prone to heat related injury, so advise your children to exercise moderately and to stop or slow down if they get short of breath. Make sure they drink plenty of fluids before, during, and after exercise. You might want to consider a liquid carbohydrate mix before your children exercise; it will keep fluid levels high and will provide plenty of energy and endurance while your child exercises. After exercise, give your children an electrolyte and carbohydrate formula to help replenish the minerals they lose in perspiration and to help restore energy levels.

One note of caution as you prepare for family fitness fun: *avoid "Little League Syndrome,"* a situation in which parents overemphasize winning and encourage children to compete beyond their emotional or physical capacity. Support your child's interests and efforts, but don't push too hard. Resist the temptation to re-live your own sports participation through your child — undue pressure on a child can cause stress, anxiety, and tension.

The key to any family fitness program is *fun.* Find activities that everyone can enjoy — and that everyone can participate in without stress, anxiety, or danger of injury. Set the example with a positive attitude toward fitness and exercise, and you'll give your children a legacy of health and fitness that will enrich their lives forever.

# Nutrition and Nutritional Supplements for Athletes

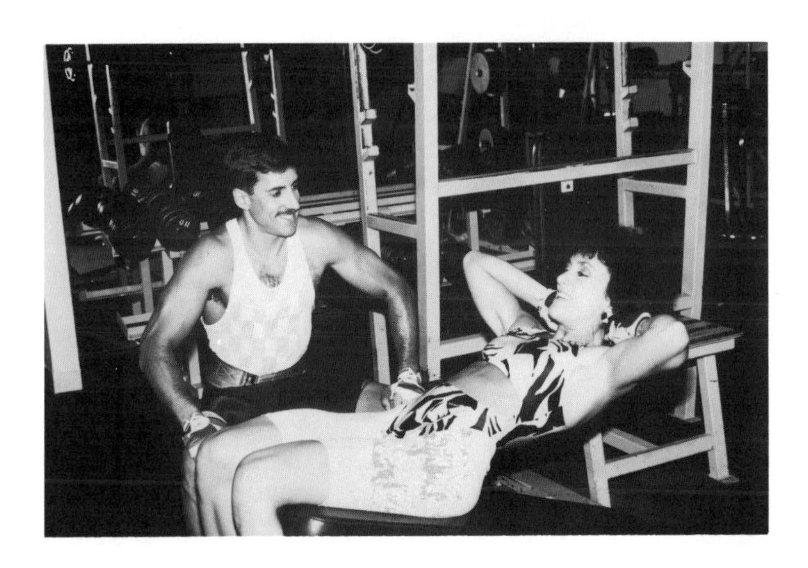

Athletes have different nutritional needs than other people?

Yes.

Then, if you're an athlete, should you disregard everything that was just discussed about nutrition?

Absolutely not! The guidelines I discussed are good, basic guidelines that serve as a foundation for people of all ages and activity levels. But because of your increased physical needs, you as an athlete will need to boost your nutritional goals in a few areas — and you'll probably need some nutritional supplements, too.

That's not all: as an athlete, you probably have weight concerns — whether you need to lose it or gain it. What follows is information tailored to you and to others who are physically active for any reason.

## Special Nutritional Needs of Athletes

Let's start at the very beginning: your basic foundation should be the nutritional plan I discussed in the previous section. Eat at least three meals a day; three to six small meals are even better. Choose low-fat, high-fiber foods from all four basic food groups so that your diet contains a good, well-balanced variety of foods. Eat most of your calories early in the day so you'll have plenty of fuel throughout the day and plenty of opportunity to burn the calories; eat fewer at night, when your body is preparing for rest. Get most of your calories from complex carbohydrates, and only 15 to 20 percent each from protein and fats.

With that foundation in place, you're ready to make the changes that athletes need: more calories, extra calories from complex carbohydrates, slightly more protein, and plenty more water.

**More Calories**

The amount of calories you need to maintain your body is determined by what's called your *basal metabolic rate.* Simply stated, it's an internal "setpoint" that is determined by your size, gender, age, percentage of body fat, and efficiency of thyroid gland function. Most people have a basal metabolic rate that requires between 1,000 and 2,000 calories per day.

When you are physically active, your calorie requirement goes up. If you are an athlete who does intensive workouts or who plays competitive sports, your basal metabolic rate will reflect your increased needs — and it may double, triple, or even quadruple over that of a moderately active person.

How can you accurately determine your calorie needs?

A physician or sports physiologist can measure your basal metabolic rate in the laboratory. There are also technical ways (such as caliper measurement and underwater submersion) to measure body fat percentage. By taking these two factors into consideration, your physician or sports physiologist can help you determine how many calories you need to maintain your present body weight — as well as how much you need if you want to gain or lose weight.

As you're consuming more calories, keep balance in mind. You should still aim for about 15 percent of your daily calories to come from protein — but you may need as much as 70 to 75 percent from carbohydrates. To avoid unnecessary increases in body fat percentages, you'll need to keep an eye on the fats you eat, too. An average diet of 2,000 calories per day can consist of 15 to 20 percent fats. When you eat 3,000 calories per day, however, your diet should be only 13.3 percent fat; at 4,000 calories, only 10 percent fat, and at 5,000 calories, only 8 percent of your daily calories should come from fats.

As an athlete, your body fat percentage needs to be lower than that of most people. A male athlete must have at least 3 percent body fat (known as "essential body fat"); young athletes should strive for a range of 5 to 12 percent, older athletes for a range of 12 to 15 percent, and athletes over 50 for a range of 15 to 20 percent.

A female athlete must have at least 10 percent body fat. Young athletes should strive for a range of 12 to 18 percent; older athletes for a range of 18 to 22 percent; and women athletes over 50 should strive for a body fat percentage of 22 to 26 percent.

If you want to maintain your present weight, use two effective tools: your bathroom scale and your own two eyes. Your weight should stay pretty even, and you should be able to see any changes in the mirror. Because of your basal metabolic rate, your body will seek to maintain *homeostasis,* or balance. Keep in mind that if your activity level increases, so will your hunger — and so will your caloric requirements.

I'll talk more later about what you can do if you want to lose weight or gain weight. For now, consider only the calories. If you want to lose, cut out 500 calories per day from your diet, and increase your activity level to burn 500 additional calories a day; a differential of 1,000 calories per day.

Since a pound of fat equals 3,500 calories, you'll expend a total of 7,000 calories — or a safe weight loss of two pounds — per week.

If you want to gain weight without gaining body fat, add 500 to 1,000 calories per day to your diet *and* make sure you exercise with weights or other resistance. It will take 2,500 extra calories to make one pound of muscle mass. Try to gain 1 to 2 pounds per week, but not more. Beyond 1 or 2 pounds and you will gain fat, not muscle!

**Carbohydrate Requirements**

As an athlete, more of your calories should come from carbohydrates — as mentioned, as much as 70 to 75 percent of your total calorie intake should be from complex carbohydrates.

You may have heard of "carbohydrate loading" — it's a technique that endurance athletes sometimes use to prepare their bodies for events. You shouldn't try carbohydrate loading on a regular basis; save it for the four to six times a year when you really need it. More often than that it's too hard on your body and, taken to an extreme, can cause your body to burn muscle tissue. Carbohydrate loading should be used only for events that exceed thirty minutes in duration; it's actually better for events that last from two to five hours.

In general, you should eat a light, high-carbohydrate meal the night before an event; rice is a good choice. On the morning of the event, eat pancakes or toast with jam or honey and a banana with several glasses of water. Make sure you get plenty of water while you are competing or exercising. You should still feel light and a little hungry before your workout — you'll have plenty of time to eat afterward.

After competition or a workout, get plenty of liquids and eat foods that are high in carbohydrates to restore needed glycogen to your muscles.

### Slight Boosts in Protein

As mentioned, protein is the subject of a fair share of nutritional myths: athletes preparing for a big event used to load up on steak and eggs in the belief that they'd enjoy greater energy. But that's not how it works; as I stated earlier, protein is a much poorer source of energy than carbohydrates. And too much of it can actually lead to toxic conditions and kidney damage.

As an athlete, you need *slightly* more protein — but take it easy! People with average activity levels should eat about .8 grams of protein per kilogram of body weight. As an athlete, you need 1 to 2 grams per kilogram of body weight. Your added requirement may be as little as 20 grams of protein — which means that you need add only have a chicken breast, a few ounces of salmon, or a few cups of yogurt to your daily diet.

Recent research shows that protein meets about 5 to 10 percent of our energy needs, and that both the liver and skeletal muscles burn protein for energy. Protein does things for you that athletes especially need — like repairing and maintaining muscle, fueling tissue growth, and synthesizing hormones.

As you add protein to your diet in small amounts, make sure

you choose low-fat sources of protein. Good sources of "lean" protein include fish, poultry (with skin removed), brown rice, low-fat dairy products, and nonfat yogurt.

**More Water**

Simply stated, water is essential to life. Lose a little bit, and your performance suffers; lose a lot, and you can die.

People with moderate activity levels need eight to ten eight-ounce glasses of water a day. You need more than that — perhaps twice as much — if you have higher activity levels or weigh more than average. During competition and during warm weather, your fluid needs increase even more.

Athletes especially need more water — and there are several reasons why. First, you're eating more protein; your body needs plenty of water to rid itself of the byproducts of protein metabolism. Unless you step up your water intake, you can suffer kidney damage from the protein you eat.

Water boosts your performance; when you start to dehydrate, you get fatigued rapidly. Too little water can cause muscle cramps. And if you get too little while exercising in warm weather, you can rapidly develop heat stroke. Athletes who get quite dehydrated during workouts are susceptible to heat stroke even indoors or in cool weather.

Even if you're trying to lose weight, drink plenty of water. Any extra will be flushed out of your body. And cut down on the amount of salt you eat: salt causes water retention and prevents perspiration, which is how your body stays cool.

How do you know if you're getting enough water?

Take a look at your urine. It should be pale yellow — about the color of lemonade. (Remember that vitamin B supplements and some medications can cause your urine to turn dark or bright yellow, however.) If your urine has a strong smell, you are probably not getting enough water.

Remember to drink plenty of water while you are exercising or competing. A good rule of thumb is to drink eight to sixteen ounces of cold water during the half hour before you begin your workout. How much you drink — and how often you drink it — during your workout depends on how long your event will last.

For events under two hours in duration, drink cold water

every fifteen minutes. For events lasting between two and five hours, drink cold water with sugar dissolved in it every fifteen minutes. Use no more than 2.5 grams of sugar per 100 ml of water; if you use juice or soft drinks, dilute them with water at a ratio of two to one (or more). *Never drink sugared water before an event;* you'll set off an insulin reaction that will cause blood sugar levels to plummet.

For events lasting more than five hours, drink sweetened water every fifteen minutes; supplement the water with easily digestible foods that are low in fats, such as bananas, rice cakes, bread with jam or honey, dates, figs, or raisins. Avoid eating proteins, which will increase your need for water. Dilute carbohydrate preparations are commercially available and work best.

After workouts, regardless of their duration, drink plenty of water. A good guideline is to drink until you are no longer thirsty — and then drink one or two more glasses. Eat foods that are high in carbohydrates to restore glycogen to the muscles, and eat some protein to help in repair and healing of muscles and tissues. For replacing the minerals lost in perspiration an electrolyte drink is preferable, which we will discuss in detail shortly.

A final note on the nutritional needs of athletes: if you do either anaerobic ar endurance exercise, you might benefit from baking soda or caffeine.

When you do anaerobic exercise (such as sprinting or lifting weights), there is often an incomplete combustion of energy sources in the muscles. As a result, the waste product from that incomplete combustion — lactic acid — builds up in the muscles, causing soreness and muscle fatigue. Sodium bicarbonate — good old baking soda — can help keep lactic acids down, delaying the onset of soreness and fatigue. Simply dissolve a heaping spoonful in water, or use a sodium bicarbonate product, such as Alka Seltzer.

If you're an endurance athlete, caffeine can help stimulate your central nervous system and can help spare glycogen, the sugar reserves stored in your muscles (and, incidentally, the best source of energy). When your glycogen stores are depleted, you "hit the wall" — or, in technical terms, your blood sugar plummets. Try drinking a cup of coffee before a competition that is more than an hour in duration.

## Winning Ways with Rice

### The food for optimum performance

Brown Rice, without question, is the world's most perfect grain. It's nutritious, inexpensive, versatile, easy to prepare, and delicious too. While brown rice is very high in energy-laden complex carbohydrates, the body's major fuel for sports and exercise related activities, it is also very low in fat, has no cholesterol, is rich in B-vitamins, and has over three times the fiber of white rice.

The key to any successful physical fitness or weight loss program is combining a well-planned exercise regimen with a solid nutritional diet. A sound nutritional program should include the following:

**3 – 5 Daily servings of**

- fruit and vegetables
- grains and cereals
- non-fat milk and non-fat dairy products
- and proteins such as fish, poultry, lean meat, eggs, legumes, and nuts

Brown rice is an optimum performance food and following are some low-calorie, low-fat, great-tasting recipes that can be used as part of your daily regimen. "Starting Line" recipes feature healthy appetizers that will quickly become favorites in your nutritional plans; "First-in-Line Favorites" has some great side-dish recipes; "Mega Results with Main Dishes" spotlights spectacular meals, some of which can be prepared in minutes; and "Finish Line Finals" highlight a host of light, refreshing desserts. These recipes feature Mahatma® Brown and Success® Brown Rice, but Mahatma® Brown Rice may be substituted with Carolina® Brown or River® Brown Rice, whichever is found at your local grocer's.

Brown rice should be an integral part of a high fuel diet for any athlete or anyone who strives for fitness.

Exercise alone is only one-half of the fitness equation. A healthy diet is equally important and brown rice should certainly be a big part of your personal Fitness Formula.

# STARTING LINE

## Seafood Primavera

| | |
|---|---|
| 2 | bags ***Success® Brown Rice*** |
| 1-1/2 | cups frozen combination vegetables; broccoli green beans, pearl onions and red peppers |
| 1/2 | cup water |
| 1 | cup skim milk OR 1 cup plain low-fat yogurt |
| 1/2 | pound imitation crab meat |
| 2 | tablespoons low-calorie margarine |
| 1 | teaspoon garlic powder |
| 3/4 | cup Parmesan cheese, grated |

Cook brown rice according to package directions.

Bring vegetables and water to a boil in a medium saucepan. Reduce heat, cover and simmer 3 minutes. Drain. Add milk or yogurt, imitation crab meat, margarine, and garlic powder. Serve on a bed of cooked brown rice. Top with Parmesan cheese.

**Serves: 4**

**1 Serving Contains:**

| | | | |
|---|---|---|---|
| Calories from Protein: | 29% | Fat — Saturated: | 4.29 g |
| Calories from Carbohydrates: | 39% | Fat — Mono: | 3.14 g |
| Calories from Fats: | 31% | Fat — Poly: | 1.72 g |
| Dietary Fiber: | 1.67 g | Cholesterol: | 57.8 mg |
| Fat — Total: | 9.81 g | Sodium: | 446 mg |

## Garden Rice Toss

| | |
|---|---|
| 1 | bag ***Success® Brown Rice*** or ***Broccoli & Cheese Rice Mix*** |
| 1 | teaspoon olive oil |
| 1 | medium onion, chopped |
| 1/2 | cup mushrooms, sliced |
| 1 | medium zucchini, sliced |
| 2 | stalks fresh broccoli, chopped |
| 15 | snow pea pods |
| 1/2 | cup kidney beans, cooked |
| 2 | teaspoons ground pepper, fresh |
| 1/3 | cup Parmesan cheese, grated |
| 3/4 | cup plain non-fat yogurt |

Cook rice according to package directions.

Heat oil in large skillet and add all vegetables and pepper, sauté until tender. Add cooked rice and toss with cheese and yogurt.

**Serves: 4**

**1 Serving Contains:**

| | | | |
|---|---|---|---|
| Calories from Protein: | 23% | Fat — Saturated: | 3.37 g |
| Calories from Carbohydrates: | 56% | Fat — Mono: | 2.56 g |
| Calories from Fats: | 22% | Fat — Poly: | 0.788 g |
| Dietary Fiber: | 7.76 g | Cholesterol: | 12.5 mg |
| Fat — Total: | 7.20 g | Sodium: | 344 mg |

## Healthy Brown Rice Salad

1 bag ***Success® Brown Rice***
1 can (16 ounce) black-eyed peas, rinse and drain
1 cup celery, chopped
1 green bell pepper, chopped
1 red bell pepper, chopped
1 clove garlic, minced
3 green onions, sliced
1 jar (4 ounce) pimientos (optional)
1/4 cup low-fat zesty Italian dressing
lettuce leaves
green olives

Cook brown rice according to package directions.

Combine all ingredients and ***gently*** toss. Marinate and chill 2 hours or longer. Garnish with lettuce and olives, if desired.

**Serves: 4**

**1 Serving Contains:**

| | | | |
|---|---|---|---|
| Calories from Protein: | 14% | Fat — Saturated: | 0.740 g |
| Calories from Carbohydrates: | 70% | Fat — Mono: | 0.906 g |
| Calories from Fats: | 16% | Fat — Poly: | 2.41 g |
| Dietary Fiber: | 11.0 g | Cholesterol: | 1.65 mg |
| Fat — Total: | 4.43 g | Sodium: | 595 mg |

## Brown Rice Tuna Mold

1 cup ***Mahatma® Brown Rice***
1 can (7 ounce) water-packed tuna, drained and flaked
1/2 cup cucumber, chopped
1/2 cup black olives, chopped
1/2 cup green onions, chopped
2 tablespoons lemon juice
1 teaspoon pepper
1 teaspoon chili powder
1 cup lite mayonnaise

Cook brown rice according to package directions.

Combine all ingredients. Press gently into a 9-inch mold or fish mold, if available. Chill for 1 hour. Remove from mold. Garnish with lemon, olives and cucumber slices.

**Serves: 6**

**1 Serving Contains:**

| | | | |
|---|---|---|---|
| Calories from Protein: | 24% | Fat — Saturated: | 0.679 g |
| Calories from Carbohydrates: | 53% | Fat — Mono | 3.16 g |
| Calories from Fats: | 23% | Fat — Poly: | 0.553 g |
| Dietary Fiber: | 2.48 g | Cholesterol: | 18.6 mg |
| Fat — Total: | 4.62 g | Sodium: | 960 mg |

## Creamy Brown Rice Soup

| | |
|---|---|
| 6 | cups low-sodium chicken stock |
| 3 | cups ***Mahatma® Brown Rice*** |
| 1 | medium onion, chopped |
| 2-1/2 | teaspoons poultry seasoning |
| 2 | boneless chicken breasts |
| 1/2 | cup low-fat milk |
| 1/2 | cup peanuts, optional |
| 1/4 | cup parsley, optional |

Bring chicken stock to a boil in medium saucepan. Add brown rice, onion, poultry seasoning and chicken. Cover and simmer 30 minutes or until rice is tender. Remove chicken and cut into strips. Stir in milk and chicken strips. Simmer 5 minutes. DO NOT BOIL.

Serve in warm bowls garnished with peanuts and fresh chopped parsley, if desired.

**Serves: 6**

**1 Serving Contains:**

| | | | |
|---|---|---|---|
| Calories from Protein: | 14% | Fat — Saturated: | 1.04 g |
| Calories from Carbohydrates: | 76% | Fat — Mono | 1.70 g |
| Calories from Fats: | 10% | Fat — Poly: | 1.30 g |
| Dietary Fiber: | 3.42 g | Cholesterol: | 4.52 g |
| Fat — Total: | 4.36 g | Sodium | 796 mg |

## FIRST IN LINE FAVORITES

### Quick Oriental Feast

1 bag ***Success® Brown Rice***
vegetable cooking spray
1/2 pound chicken strips
2 cups mushrooms, fresh, sliced
6 green onions, chopped
1 can (8 ounce) water chestnuts, sliced
1 package (10 ounce) frozen pea pods, thawed and drained
2 teaspoons cornstarch
1/2 cup chicken broth, low sodium
2 teaspoon soy sauce, light (optional)

Cook brown rice according to package directions.

Spray skillet with vegetable cooking spray. Stir-fry chicken until lightly browned. Remove from pan and spray again with vegetable cooking spray. Heat. Add mushrooms, green onions, water chestnuts, and pea pods. Sauté until tender. Combine cornstarch, chicken broth and soy sauce (optional). Mix well and add to chicken-vegetable mixture. Allow to simmer until thickened.

Serve over hot, cooked brown rice.

**Serves: 4**

**1 Serving Contains:**

| | | | |
|---|---|---|---|
| Calories from Protein: | 30% | Fat — Saturated: | 1.42 g |
| Calories from Carbohydrates: | 55% | Fat — Mono: | 1.88 g |
| Calories from Fats: | 15% | Fat — Poly: | 1.48 g |
| Dietary Fiber: | 7.39 g | Cholesterol: | 50.6 mg |
| Fat — Total: | 5.57 g | Sodium: | 222 mg |

### Country Stew

2 bags ***Success® Brown Rice***
1 pound lean ground turkey
1 small onion, chopped
1/2 teaspoon basil
1/2 teaspoon garlic powder
2 cans (16 ounce) tomatoes, chopped
1 teaspoon pepper
1 can (16 ounce) corn

Cook brown rice according to package directions.

Brown ground turkey with onion. Add basil and garlic powder. Add tomatoes and pepper; simmer 20 minutes. Add corn and cooked brown rice. Mix. Heat thoroughly.

**Serves: 6-8**

**1 Serving Contains:**

| | | | |
|---|---|---|---|
| Calories from Protein: | 24% | Fat — Saturated: | 2.44 g |
| Calories from Carbohydrates: | 49% | Fat — Mono: | 3.38 g |
| Calories from Fats: | 27% | Fat — Poly: | 2.58 g |
| Dietary Fiber: | 3.89 g | Cholesterol: | 39.1 mg |
| Fat — Total: | 9.58 g | Sodium: | 198 mg |

## Sautéed Chicken with Brown Rice

| | |
|---|---|
| 2 | bags ***Success® Brown Rice*** |
| 1 | tablespoon vegetable oil |
| 1/4 | cup flour |
| 1/2 | teaspoon paprika |
| 1/4 | teaspoon pepper |
| 2 | cups chicken, cooked |
| 1 | medium onion, sliced |
| 1 | green pepper, chopped |
| 1 | jar (14 ounce) mushrooms, sliced and drained |
| 1/4 | cup apple juice |
| 2 | tablespoons brown sugar |

Cook brown rice according to package directions.

While rice is cooking, heat oven to 425°. Heat oil in 13x9x2 inch baking dish. Mix flour, paprika and pepper. Coat chicken with flour mixture. Place chicken in baking dish. Bake covered 30 minutes.

Remove chicken, drain fat from baking dish. Place cooked rice in dish. Arrange onion, green pepper, and mushrooms in dish. Arrange chicken on vegetables. Mix apple juice and brown sugar. Pour over chicken. Cover. Bake 20 to 30 minutes.

May be garnished with orange slices.

**Serves: 6 to 8**

**1 Serving Contains:**

| | | | |
|---|---|---|---|
| Calories from Protein | 27% | Fat — Saturated: | 0.653 g |
| Calories from Carbohydrates: | 61% | Fat — Mono: | 0.870 g |
| Calories from Fats: | 11% | Fat — Poly: | 0.770 g |
| Dietary Fiber: | 3.12 g | Cholesterol: | 29.5 mg |
| Fat — Total: | 2.69 g | Sodium: | 245 mg |

## Traditional Fried Rice with Turkey and Pine Nuts

1 bag ***Success® Brown Rice***
1 tablespoon salad oil
1 small onion, chopped
1 medium bell pepper, diced
1/4 pound mushrooms, sliced
1/4 pound turkey, cooked and cubed
1/4 cup pine nuts, roasted
2 tablespoons light soy sauce (optional)
green onions, sliced to garnish

Cook brown rice according to package directions. Refrigerate.

Place wok or frying pan over medium heat, add oil. Add onion, sauté until tender. Remove from pan and set aside.

Sauté bell pepper and mushrooms until tender. Add cooked rice, turkey, pine nuts and soy sauce, if desired.

Toss gently. Garnish with green onions.

**Serves: 6**

**1 Serving Contains:**

| | | | |
|---|---|---|---|
| Calories from Protein: | 20% | Fat — Saturated: | 2.47 g |
| Calories from Carbohydrates: | 30% | Fat — Mono: | 6.49 g |
| Calories from Fats: | 50% | Fat — Poly: | 5.65 g |
| Dietary Fiber: | 2.23 g | Cholesterol: | 13.1 mg |
| Fat — Total: | 15.5 g | Sodium: | 17.5 mg |

## Shrimp Stir Fry

1 bag ***Success® Brown Rice***
cooking spray
3 carrots, sliced
1 medium bell pepper, cut in strips
1 tablespoon corn starch
2 – 3 tablespoons lite soy sauce
3/4 pound cleaned, cooked shrimp (or any other cooked meat)
1 carton (6 ounce) low-fat yogurt
8 ounces pea pods

Cook brown rice according to package directions.

Spray skillet or wok with vegetable spray. Add carrots and peppers. Stir fry until tender. Mix cornstarch and soy sauce. Add to vegetables. Heat until thickened. Remove from heat. Stir in shrimp or other meat, yogurt and pea pods. Heat through for about 5 minutes. Serve over cooked brown rice.

**Serves: 6**

**1 Serving Contains:**

| | | | |
|---|---|---|---|
| Calories from Protein: | 35% | Fat — Saturated: | 0.613 g |
| Calories from Carbohydrates: | 56% | Fat — Mono: | 0.488 g |
| Calories from Fats: | 10% | Fat — Poly: | 0.689 g |
| Dietary Fiber: | 3.98 g | Cholesterol: | 87.9 mg |
| Fat — Total: | 2.14 g | Sodium: | 300 mg |

## Fried Rice with Bacon, Lettuce and Tomato

1 cup ***Mahatma® Brown Rice***
4 slices turkey bacon
1/4 cup onions, chopped
1 teaspoon sherry, optional
2 tablespoons low-sodium chicken broth
1 cup lettuce, shredded
1 tomato, cut in strips, pulp and seeds removed
1 teaspoon Worcestershire sauce (optional)

Cook rice according to package directions. Refrigerate until cool.

Cook turkey bacon in wok. Fry until crisp. Remove turkey bacon, drain on paper towel and crumble. Remove all fat from wok. Increase heat to medium.

Add onions and stir-fry about 1 minute. Add sherry and chicken broth. Place cooked rice on top. Cover and steam for 30-seconds. Uncover and stir-fry until rice is hot. Stir in lettuce and tomato strips and crumbled turkey bacon. Sprinkle with Worcestershire sauce, if desired. Stir-fry until well-blended.

**Serves: 6**

**1 Serving Contains:**

| | | | |
|---|---|---|---|
| Calories from Protein: | 14% | Fat — Saturated: | 0.135 g |
| Calories from Carbohydrates: | 68% | Fat — Mono | 0.230 g |
| Calories from Fats: | 18% | Fat — Poly: | 0.264 g |
| Dietary Fiber: | 1.77 g | Cholesterol: | .007 mg |
| Fat — Total: | 2.06 g | Sodium: | 7.81 mg |

## MEGA RESULTS WITH MAIN DISHES

## Mexican Rice Ole!

2 bags ***Success® Brown Rice***
1 tablespoon low-calorie margarine
1/2 cup onion, finely chopped
1/2 teaspoon garlic powder
1 can (5.8 ounce) whole kernel corn, drained
3/4 cup non-fat yogurt
1/2 cup lite Cheddar cheese, shredded
1 small can (4 ounce) green chilies, chopped

Cook brown rice according to package directions.

Place margarine in skillet. Sauté onions. Add garlic powder and corn. Add cooked rice. Fold in remaining ingredients. Heat.

**Serves: 4 to 6**

**1 Serving Contains:**

| | | | |
|---|---|---|---|
| Calories from Protein: | 23% | Fat — Saturated: | 4.53 g |
| Calories from Carbohydrates: | 51% | Fat — Mono: | 0.855 g |
| Calories from Fats: | 26% | Fat — Poly: | 0.842 g |
| Dietary Fiber: | 3.12 g | Cholesterol: | 27.5 mg |
| Fat — Total: | 9.09 g | Sodium: | 424 mg |

## Romanoff Rice

1 bag ***Success® Brown Rice***
1 teaspoon margarine
8 ounces fresh mushrooms, sliced
1 cup non-fat yogurt
1/2 teaspoon pepper
1/2 teaspoon garlic powder
Parmesan cheese

Cook brown rice according to package directions.

Melt margarine in a skillet. Sauté mushrooms. Add cooked rice, non-fat yogurt, pepper and garlic powder. Spoon mixture into a small, oiled, baking dish, sprinkle with cheese. Cover and bake 20 minutes at 350°.

**Serves: 4 to 6**

**1 Serving Contains:**

| | | | |
|---|---|---|---|
| Calories from Protein: | 11% | Fat — Saturated: | 0.761 g |
| Calories from Carbohydrates: | 76% | Fat — Mono: | 1.37 g |
| Calories from Fats: | 13% | Fat — Poly: | 1.53 g |
| Dietary Fiber: | 2.83 g | Cholesterol: | .667 mg |
| Fat — Total: | 3.94 g | Sodium: | 60.3 mg |

## Savory Cornish Hens with Herbed Rice

2 Cornish game hens, thawed
2 tablespoons low-calorie margarine, softened
1/2 cup dry white wine, divided
1/4 cup green onions, sliced
1 garlic clove, minced
1 teaspoon marjoram leaves
1/4 teaspoon pepper
1 can (10-1/2 ounce) low-sodium chicken broth, divided
1 cup ***Mahatma® Brown Rice***
1 cup mushrooms, sliced

Remove giblets from hens. With sharp knife, cut hens in half lengthwise. Loosen skin from meat on breast of each half to form pocket; place in shallow baking dish.

Cream margarine and add 2 tablespoons of the wine, green onions, garlic, marjoram, and pepper. Mix well. Spoon about a teaspoon of the margarine mixture into pocket of each hen half. Pour 1/2 cup chicken broth over hens. Cover and bake at 350° basting occasionally with the drippings, for 30 minutes. Remove cover and bake another 30 minutes.

While hens are baking, add enough water to remaining broth to make 2 cups.

Pour into 3-quart saucepan. Add remaining wine and margarine mixture. Bring to a boil. Stir in brown rice and mushrooms. Cover and simmer over moderately low heat for 45 minutes.

Serve hen halves over the rice.

**Serves: 6**

**1 Serving Contains:**

| | | | |
|---|---|---|---|
| Calories from Protein: | 40% | Fat — Saturated: | 1.49 g |
| Calories from Carbohydrates: | 39% | Fat — Mono: | 2.23 g |
| Calories from Fats: | 22% | Fat — Poly: | 1.72 g |
| Dietary Fiber: | 1.41 g | Cholesterol: | 58.0 mg |
| Fat — Total: | 6.23 g | Sodium: | 211 mg |

## Vegetarian Brown Rice Salad

- 1 cup ***Mahatma ® Brown Rice***
- 3/4 cup scallions
- 1/4 cup snow pea pods, blanched
- 3/4 cup celery, chopped
- 1 medium cucumber, diced
- 1/2 cup radishes, sliced
- 2 tablespoons red peppers, chopped
- 2 tablespoons fresh parsley, minced
- 1-1/2 tablespoons rice vinegar
- 1 teaspoon lemon juice
- 1 teaspoon lite soy sauce
- 1 teaspoon pepper
- 1 teaspoon paprika
- 2 tablespoons safflower oil

Cook brown rice according to package directions. Cool.

Combine cooked rice, scallions, pea pods, celery, cucumbers, radishes, red peppers, and parsley in a large bowl. Place vinegar, lemon juice, soy sauce, pepper, and paprika in a small bowl. Add oil gradually, beating constantly with a wire whisk until blended. Pour over rice and vegetables. Toss and combine.

Chill at least 2 hours.

**Serves: 10**

**1 Serving Contains:**

| | | | |
|---|---|---|---|
| Calories from Protein: | 8% | Fat — Saturated: | 0.345 g |
| Calories from Carbohydrates: | 57% | Fat — Mono: | 0.471 g |
| Calories from Fats: | 36% | Fat — Poly: | 2.21 g |
| Dietary Fiber: | 1.86 g | Cholesterol: | 0 mg |
| Fat — Total: | 3.30 g | Sodium: | 68.5 mg |

## Chicken and Broccoli Rice Supreme

1-1/2 cup ***Mahatma® Brown Rice***
1/2 cup onions, chopped
1/2 cup mushrooms, sliced
1 tablespoon low-calorie margarine
1 cup chicken, cooked, diced
1 package (10 ounce) frozen broccoli, thawed and drained
1 can (10-3/4 ounce) condensed cream of mushroom soup, low-sodium
1 jar (2 ounce) pimientos
1/2 cup low-fat Cheddar cheese, shredded

Cook brown rice according to package directions.

Sauté onions and mushrooms in margarine in a skillet until tender. Stir in cooked rice, chicken, broccoli, soup and pimientos. Pour into greased shallow 1-1/2 quart baking dish. Top with cheese. Bake at 350° for 20 minutes.

**Serves: 6**

**1 Serving Contains:**

| | | | |
|---|---|---|---|
| Calories from Protein: | 18% | Fat — Saturated: | 5.40 g |
| Calories from Carbohydrates: | 63% | Fat — Mono: | 2.30 g |
| Calories from Fats: | 19% | Fat — Poly: | 2.19 g |
| Dietary Fiber: | 9.99 g | Cholesterol: | 44.9 mg |
| Fat — Total: | 16.4 g | Sodium: | 566 mg |

## Creole Chicken

1 tablespoon corn oil
1 cup onion, chopped
2 cups green pepper, chopped
3 tablespoons parsley, chopped
1 garlic clove, minced
1 can (16 ounce) stewed tomatoes
3 cups low-sodium chicken stock
1/4 teaspoon basil
1/2 teaspoon thyme
1/4 teaspoon cayenne pepper
2 bay leaves
1-1/2 cup ***Mahatma® Brown Rice***
2 cups chicken, cooked and cubed
1 cup lean ham, cubed

Heat oil in skillet. Sauté onion, green pepper, parsley, and garlic. Add tomatoes and cook for 2 minutes. Add chicken stock, basil, thyme, cayenne, and bay leaves. Bring to a boil. Stir in brown rice. Reduce heat and cover. Simmer 30 to 40 minutes. Add chicken and ham. Heat thoroughly and remove bay leaves.

**Serves: 6**

**1 Serving Contains:**

| | | | |
|---|---|---|---|
| Calories from Protein: | 27% | Fat — Saturated | 1.91 g |
| Calories from Carbohydrates: | 52% | Fat — Mono: | 2.80 g |
| Calories from Fats: | 21% | Fat — Poly: | 2.81 g |
| Dietary Fiber: | 4.17 g | Cholesterol: | 50.8 mg |
| Fat — Total: | 8.77 g | Sodium: | 441 mg |

## Curried Beef and Brown Rice

- 1/2 pound lean ground chicken or ground turkey
- 1 cup onions, chopped
- 2 cups low-sodium beef broth
- 1 can (4 ounce) mushrooms, drained
- 1 teaspoon curry powder
- 1 teaspoon Worcestershire sauce (optional)
- 1 cup ***Mahatma® Brown Rice***
- 1 can (16 ounce) whole green beans, drained

Brown ground chicken in a skillet. Add onions and next 5 ingredients. Bring to a boil. Add brown rice. Cover and reduce heat. Simmer 35 minutes or until rice is done. Add green beans and toss.

**Serves: 4 to 6**

**1 Serving Contains:**

| | | | |
|---|---|---|---|
| Calories from Protein: | 30% | Fat — Saturated: | 0.698 g |
| Calories from Carbohydrates: | 57% | Fat — Mono: | 0.965 g |
| Calories from Fats: | 13% | Fat — Poly: | 0.774 g |
| Dietary Fiber: | 3.00 g | Cholesterol: | 31.9 mg |
| Fat — Total: | 3.10 g | Sodium: | 326 mg |

## Spanish Brown Rice Dinner

- 3 cups ***Mahatma® Brown Rice***
- 1 cup onions, chopped
- 1 can (4 ounce) green chilies, chopped and drained
- 1/2 teaspoon ground cumin
- 1/2 teaspoon Italian seasoning
- 1 can (15 ounce) tomato sauce
- 1/2 cup low-sodium chicken broth
- 1 cup chicken, cooked and diced
- 1 cup non-fat yogurt
- 1 cup low-fat Cheddar cheese, shredded
- 1 cup corn chips, crushed (optional)

Cook brown rice according to package directions.

Combine onions, chilies, cumin, Italian seasoning, tomato sauce, and broth in a saucepan. Cover and simmer for 15 minutes. Add chicken; set aside. Combine cooked rice and yogurt in a baking dish. Sprinkle with Cheddar cheese. Bake uncovered at 350° for 10 minutes. Sprinkle with corn chips.

**Serves: 6**

**1 Serving Contains:**

| | | | |
|---|---|---|---|
| Calories from Protein: | 28% | Fat — Saturated: | 8.79 g |
| Calories from Carbohydrates: | 44% | Fat — Mono: | 1.01 g |
| Calories from Fats: | 28% | Fat — Poly: | 0.943 g |
| Dietary Fiber: | 5.13 g | Cholesterol: | 194 mg |
| Fat — Total: | 16.7 g | Sodium: | 654 mg |

## Tuna, Veggies and Brown Rice

1 cup ***Mahatma® Brown Rice***
4 ounces Monterrey Jack cheese, cut in strips
1 large zucchini, sliced
1 cup tomato, chopped
1 cup non-fat yogurt
1 can (4 ounce) green chilies, chopped and drained
1/4 cup onion, chopped
3/4 teaspoon garlic powder
1 medium tomato, sliced

Cook brown rice according to package directions.

Heat oven to 350°. Reserve 1/4 of cheese strips. Layer 1/2 of rice, cheese, zucchini, and chopped tomato in an ungreased 2-quart casserole. Repeat layers.

Mix yogurt, chilies, onion and garlic powder. Spread over vegetable rice mixture. Arrange sliced tomato on yogurt mixture. Top with reserved cheese strips. Bake uncovered for 20 minutes.

**Serves: 8**

**1 Serving Contains:**

| | | | |
|---|---|---|---|
| Calories from Protein: | 21% | Fat — Saturated: | 1.71 g |
| Calories from Carbohydrates: | 60% | Fat — Mono: | 0.286 g |
| Calories from Fats: | 19% | Fat — Poly: | 0.313 g |
| Dietary Fiber: | 1.65 g | Cholesterol: | 10.6 mg |
| Fat — Total: | 3.42 g | Sodium: | 139 mg |

# FINISH LINE FINALS

## Cran-Berry Delight

1 bag ***Success® Brown Rice***
1 can (8 ounce) whole cranberry jelly (or any whole berry jelly or preserve)
1 can (15-1/4 ounce) pineapple chunks, drained
1/2 cup pecans, chopped
1 carton (3 ounce) low-fat vanilla yogurt
1 package sugar-free orange gelatin
1 cup hot water

Cook brown rice according to package directions.

*As a Sauce:* Combine first four ingredients. Heat slightly and serve over brown rice.

*As a Salad:* Combine all ingredients. Pour into a mold. Chill and serve.

**Serves: 4**

**1 Serving Contains:**

| | | | |
|---|---|---|---|
| Calories from Protein: | 7% | Fat — Saturated: | 0.796 g |
| Calories from Carbohydrates: | 75% | Fat — Mono: | 3.60 g |
| Calories from Fats: | 18% | Fat — Poly: | 1.78 g |
| Dietary Fiber: | 5.19 g | Cholesterol: | 1.07 mg |
| Fat — Total: | 6.72 g | Sodium: | 38.3 mg |

## Apple and Brown Rice Pudding

1 cup ***Mahatma® Brown Rice***
2-1/2 cups water
2-1/2 cups skim milk, divided
3 egg whites
1/2 cup sugar
2 large apples, peeled, cored and coarsely chopped
1/2 cup dark seedless grapes
1/2 cup dried apricots, quartered
2 tablespoons vanilla extract

In a heavy 4-quart saucepan, heat water to boiling. Stir in rice. Cover and cook over low heat for 20 minutes.

Add 2 cups milk to partially cooked rice, stirring occasionally to prevent sticking. Cook about 20 minutes longer or until rice is tender.

In a small bowl, with a wire whisk, beat together remaining milk and eggs whites. Stir in sugar, add apples, grapes, apricots and vanilla. Cook , stirring constantly, until mixture thickens. (DO NOT BOIL.)

**Serves: 8**

**1 Serving Contains:**

| | | | |
|---|---|---|---|
| Calories from Protein: | 10% | Fat — Saturated: | 0.933 g |
| Calories from Carbohydrates: | 81% | Fat — Mono: | 0.643 g |
| Calories from Fats: | 9% | Fat — Poly: | 0.361 g |
| Dietary Fiber: | 2.61 g | Cholesterol: | 5.50 mg |
| Fat — Total: | 2.17 g | Sodium: | 60.4 mg |

## Blueberry Brown Rice Crisp

3/4 cup ***Mahatma® Brown Rice***
3 cups blueberries
2 tablespoons lemon juice
2/3 cup packed brown sugar
1/2 cup flour
1/4 cup margarine, softened
3/4 tablespoon ground cinnamon
whipped topping

Cook brown rice according to package directions.

While rice is cooking, heat oven to 350°. Place blueberries in an ungreased square baking dish. Sprinkle with lemon juice. Mix brown sugar, flour, brown rice, margarine and cinnamon. Sprinkle on top of blueberries. Bake until topping is light brown, about 15 minutes. Serve warm with whipped topping.

**Serves: 6**

**1 Serving Contains:**

| | | | |
|---|---|---|---|
| Calories from Protein: | 4% | Fat — Saturated: | 0.810 g |
| Calories from Carbohydrates: | 81% | Fat — Mono: | 1.66 g |
| Calories from Fats: | 15% | Fat — Poly: | 1.60 g |
| Dietary Fiber: | 2.73 g | Cholesterol: | 0 mg |
| Fat — Total: | 4.29 g | Sodium: | 18.2 mg |

## Fruit Tart

**Crust**

| | |
|---|---|
| 1 | cup ***Mahatma® Brown Rice*** |
| 1/4 | cup sugar |
| 2 | egg whites, beaten |
| 1 | teaspoon cinnamon |

Cook brown rice according to package directions.

In a mixing bowl, combine cooked rice with remaining ingredients. Press into a 8-inch springform pan. Bake 350° for 10 minutes. Cool to room temperature.

**Filling**

| | |
|---|---|
| 2 | packages (8 ounce) lite cream cheese |
| 1/2 | cup non-fat yogurt |
| 1/2 | cup confectioners sugar |
| 2 | teaspoons vanilla |

Combine cream cheese and non-fat yogurt in a medium bowl until light and fluffy. Add sugar and vanilla. Blend. Spread over cooled brown rice crust. Refrigerate until cream mixture has set.

**Topping**

| | |
|---|---|
| | sliced fresh fruit |
| 1/2 | cup apple jelly |

Arrange sliced fresh fruit on top of cooled, cream mixture. Heat apple jelly until dissolved. Brush on top of fruit.

**Serves: 8 (1 pie)**

**1 Serving Contains:**

| | | | |
|---|---|---|---|
| Calories from Protein: | 11% | Fat — Saturated: | 8.17 g |
| Calories from Carbohydrates: | 45% | Fat — Mono: | 0.093 g |
| Calories from Fats: | 43% | Fat — Poly: | 0.086 g |
| Dietary Fiber: | 0.592 g | Cholesterol: | 50.9 mg |
| Fat — Total: | 14.4 g | Sodium | 263 mg |

## Rice'n Peaches 'n Cream

| | |
|---|---|
| 1 | cup ***Mahatma® Brown Rice*** |
| 1 | can (16 ounce) peaches, sliced |
| 1/3 | cup brown sugar |
| 1 | tablespoon margarine |
| 1 | teaspoon lemon juice |
| 1/4 | teaspoon ground cinnamon |
| 1/4 | teaspoon nutmeg |
| 1/2 | cup whipped topping |

Cook brown rice according to package directions.

Drain peaches and reserve 1/2 cup of the liquid and about 12 of the peach slices. Dice remaining peaches.

Stir the chopped peaches, reserved peach liquid, brown sugar, margarine, lemon juice, cinnamon, and nutmeg into hot cooked rice. Mix well, simmer 5 minutes.

Pour into buttered 1-1/2 quart casserole. Pour the whipped topping over the rice. Arrange the remaining peaches over the top.

Bake at 450° for 15 minutes.

**Serves: 6**

**1 Serving Contains:**

| | | | |
|---|---|---|---|
| Calories from Protein: | 4% | Fat — Saturated: | 4.24 g |
| Calories from Carbohydrates: | 74% | Fat — Mono: | 2.53 g |
| Calories from Fats: | 22% | Fat — Poly: | 0.836 g |
| Dietary Fiber: | 2.16 g | Cholesterol: | 22.1 mg |
| Fat — Total: | 8.04 g | Sodium | 47.8 mg |

## Cooking Tips for Mahatma® Brown, Carolina® Brown, River® Brown or Success® Brown Rice

*1. Shorten your Mahatma® Brown Rice cooking time by soaking brown rice in water for up to a 4-hour period. Drain the liquid and measure. Then add enough water to equal the amount needed to cook the rice. (2-1/2 cups water for 1 cup dry rice). Cook only 20 minutes!

*2. Microwave your Mahatma® Brown Rice! For microwave cooking use only 2 cups liquid per 1 cup uncooked brown rice. Combine the water, rice, salt and margarine in a 2 to 3 quart casserole dish. Cover and cook on ***high*** (100%) for 5- minutes. Reduce power to 30% and cook 45 minutes.

3. Substitute cooked brown rice in any recipe calling for cooked rice. A pleasing way to add fiber to your diet. Brown rice is one of nature's few foods that contains all of the major nutrient groups.
4. Brown rice is high in natural dietary fiber. Medical research has found that dietary fiber is an important factor for good health.
5. Try tossing cooked brown rice with light soy sauce or teriyaki sauce. Add your favorite Chinese vegetable! A quick, easy and low fat meal.
6. A salad for all seasons: cooled brown rice tossed with any chopped, seasonal vegetables and your favorite low calorie dressing makes an excellent high fiber, low calorie meal.
7. In 2 tablespoons of butter or margarine, sauté 1 jar (2-1/2 ounces) sliced mushrooms, drained and 1/4 cup sliced green onions. Stir into cooked brown rice.
8. Combine 3 cups cooked brown rice with 2 tablespoons butter or margarine, 1 packet instant chicken broth and 1 teaspoon parsley flakes for a delicious chicken-seasoned flavored rice.
9. Combine 1/2 cup milk, 1/2 cup shredded cheese and 1 packet instant broth. Heat until cheese melts. Stir in 3 cups of cooked, hot brown rice for a cheesy rice dish.
10. Combine 3 cups cooked brown rice with 2 cups water, 4 packets instant onion broth, 1 tablespoon butter or margarine, and 1 teaspoon Worcestershire sauce. Heat thoroughly for a great onion rice soup.
11. Pepperoni, artichoke hearts, mozzarella cheese, olives, and chilled cooked brown rice with a tomato-based dressing create the perfect Italian Salad.
12. For Waldorf salad, add to chilled cooked brown rice, raisins, red apples, walnuts, celery and light low-cholesterol mayonnaise.
13. Add your favorite spaghetti sauce and Parmesan cheese to cooked brown rice for a delicious Italian dinner.
14. For quick jambalaya, try adding cooked brown rice to stewed tomatoes, smoked turkey and Cajun seasoning.
15. Almonds, dates and honey added to cooked brown rice make a great combination snack.

*** Mahatma® Brown Rice may be substituted with Carolina® Brown or River® Brown Rice.**

## Nutritional Supplements for Athletes

Just as athletes have some increased need for certain nutrients, they also need nutritional supplementation that moderately active people don't necessarily require.

When you think of "nutritional supplements," the first things that come to mind are probably daily vitamin capsules. But when you exercise, you need to deliver oxygen and fuel to your working muscles. As you continue to exercise, you need to replenish the water and electrolytes that you sweat away. You get oxygen from the air you breathe — but you have to consume the water, fuel, and electrolytes. The harder you exercise, the more important these "supplements" are if you want to counter the heavy demands you're placing on your body.

As an athlete, you should consider a good carbohydrate supplement, a comprehensive vitamin/mineral supplement, herbal supplements to enhance energy, and an electrolyte replacement drink.

### Carbohydrate Supplement

What are the fuels of choice during exercise?

Forget about the simple sugars — you know, the kind found in candy bars. Why? They are metabolized quickly, get into your system rapidly, and cause a big burst of energy. What's so bad about that? The crash that follows. As simple sugars course through your bloodstream, your pancreas begins pumping out insulin to counter the increase in blood sugar. As a result, your system in overloaded with insulin, your blood sugar drops dramatically, and you "hit the wall."

The fuel of choice during exercise, then, are complex carbohydrates — those that break down more slowly and provide a sustained flow of energy. As you exercise, your body burns glycogen stored in your muscles and liver; as exercise continues, your body also begins burning store fat.

What happens then?

Everything's fine, as long as you don't run out of stored glycogen. When you do run out out stored glycogen, *even if you still have plenty of stored fat to burn,* you crash. Why? Because fat only burns if it has a glycogen wick. If there's no carbohydrate present during exercise, fats aren't utilized.

That's not all. When you run out of stored glycogen, you feel fatigued, weak, and dizzy. If you hope to continue your workout, you need to replace your glycogen quickly and efficiently. To do it, the best way is to combine a highly digestible carbohydrate source with water — and to use it before, during, and after your workout.

I've found that a good carbohydrate sports drink powder is best to use — and the best kind of powder is one that contains both simple and complex carbohydrates. Carbohydrate sports drink powders are good choices because they assimilate into the body quickly, they are easy and convenient to use, and they can be placed in a water bottle for convenient use during a workout.

**Vitamin/Mineral Supplements**

Athletes and other physically active people have special vitamin and mineral needs because of the physiological changes the body undergoes during exercise. As an example, both the B-complex vitamins (necessary for carbohydrate digestion) and vitamin C are lost through heavy perspiration. Athletes also need extra magnesium, calcium, zinc, potassium, and iron; women athletes have a particularly critical need for increased calcium and iron to prevent osteoporosis and anemia.

As mentioned earlier, a vitamin/mineral supplement should be used as an "insurance policy" against possible malnutrition, but should *never be used to replace food in your diet.*

Choose a good vitamin/mineral supplement that provides 100 percent of the recommended daily allowance of the nutrients athletes need most.

**Herbs for Energy**

A number of herbal supplements and other food supplements may provide you with the energy and stamina that are beneficial to athletes. At various times during my professional career, I have taken certain herbs, ergogenic aids, and food supplements for the benefits they may give. Some of these have included bee pollen, brewer's yeast, octacosanol, lecithin, choline, inositol, zinc, and ginseng.

There are a number of herbal formulas on the market that can help increase muscle mass, provide energy, boost endurance, and enhance the body's ability to withstand stress — all without the adverse side effects of steroids and other medications.

**Electrolyte Replacement Drink**

When you have finished working out, you need to replace the water you have lost through perspiration. But that's not all: you need to begin replacing water during your workout as well, especially if your workout exceeds thirty minutes in duration.

That sounds easy — just drink water, right?

Unfortunately, it's not that simple. The water or other fluid that you drink during a workout will do you no good if it stays in your stomach; to be effective in preventing dehydration, it needs to leave your stomach quickly and be rapidly absorbed by your cells. I'll never forget an Ironman Triathlon competitor who *gained* more than ten pounds during her race because of all the water she drank — but who became severely dehydrated. How could someone possibly become dehydrated after swilling *ten pounds of water?* Simple: it stayed in her stomach.

Fortunately, the solution is an easy one. Isotonic electrolyte solutions are absorbed much more rapidly than water; these solutions leave your stomach quickly and are absorbed by your body cells, where they are needed to overcome the danger of dehydration during workouts. There's another advantage to electrolyte solutions over water: because they are absorbed more quickly, you won't have to drink as much. And the obvious final advantage is that they replace the electrolytes lost in perspiration — so, unlike water, they are great to use at the end of your workout.

One caution: steer clear of electrolyte replacement drinks that contain too much sugar and sodium, such as Gatorade®. When sugar and sodium are present in heavy concentrations, the electrolyte solution is actually absorbed by the body more slowly than plain water.

In addition to using a good isotonic electrolyte replacement drink, I like to use Siberian ginseng after my workouts. Why? The Soviets refer to Siberian ginseng as an "adaptogen" because it helps the body adapt to physical stress and strain. Athletes worldwide have begun using Siberian ginseng not only to enhance performance, but to cut down recovery time after workouts.

# Becoming a Lean Machine: How to Lose Weight Effectively

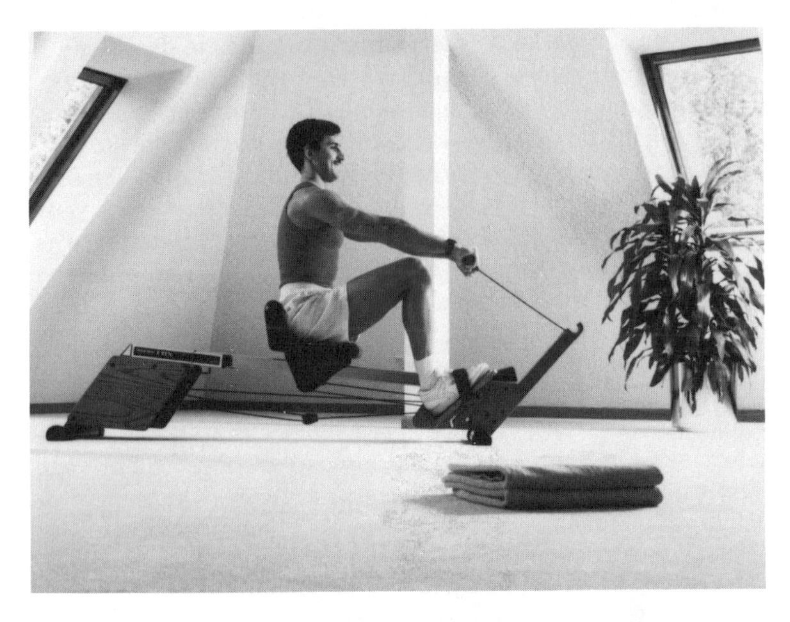

To begin any discussion about weight loss, it seems necessary to state the obvious: muscle is muscle , and fat is adipose tissue. Fat will never turn to muscle, and muscle will never turn to fat. Fat comes from the foods you have eaten that your body didn't need for fuel; your body stored it for later use. The fat will be burned when your body needs it — and that's only when there's not another energy source available.

I've already outlined the basics of losing weight: *intelligently* cut back of the food you eat and step up the amount of exercise you get. Fat loss isn't accomplished by diet alone or by exercise alone — it takes time and hard work, and it requires an effective combination of both diet and exercise.

**Diet**

I listed some excellent nutritional guidelines in the first section of this book; read them over again. If you need to lose weight, remember that the biggest enemy in your diet is *fat.* It does more than just make you obese — it has been definitely linked to cardiovascular disease, atherosclerosis, cancer (especially of the breast and colon), hemorrhoids, and constipation.

Unfortunately, fat tastes good. And, because it takes so long to digest, it is satisfying. If you're used to eating a diet rich in fatty foods, you'll have to make some changes if you want to lose weight.

A basic weight-loss diet should consist primarily of complex carbohydrates — fruits, vegetables, starches, breads, rice, potatoes, and whole-grain cereals. They are the body's best source of energy, they are low in fat, and they are rich in fiber. You should get at least 60 percent of your calories from complex carbohydrates; as an athlete, you will probably need closer to 70 or 75 percent because you'll need the extra fuel during workouts.

If you don't have a taste for carbohydrate-rich foods, develop one. It's the best thing you can do for your body! You wouldn't expect a sleek, cherry-red Ferrari to run on watered-down gasoline and oil; don't expect your body to perform well when it's been fueled by Twinkies.

The remaining 20 percent or so of your diet should consist of high-quality, lean protein foods, such as fish, poultry without skin, egg whites, and skim dairy products.

Remember to drink plenty of water. Protein increases your need for water, as discussed, and so do carbohydrates. Water is especially important when you are trying to lose weight — so drink at least ten eight-ounce glasses every day, and more when you are working out.

The foods you eat — even when they are lean — contain all the fat you need in your diet. A good rule of thumb when trying to lose weight is to *never consciously add fat to your diet.* That means skipping butter. Salad dressing. Cream in your coffee. Mayonnaise on your sandwich.

Sound impossible?

It's not! Use your imagination — you can come up with plenty of "tricks" to compensate for the fact that you're cutting out fats. Sprinkle herbs and spices on your steamed vegetables instead of slathering them with butter; instead of heaping butter and sour cream on a baked potato, try a topping of nonfat yogurt or cottage cheese. Try vinegar or lemon juice (or a combination) on your salads. Instead of butter on your toast, try sugar-free jam or honey. Use egg whites and vegetables with rice, cooked in a non-stick pan to make fried rice without the oil and fat.

Limit your use of eggs — and when you do use them, cut out

the yolks where possible. Many recipes work out fine if you substitute two egg whites for one egg; when making scrambled eggs or omelets, use one yolk per serving and make up the bulk of the dish with egg whites.

Be conscious of how you prepare your foods. In general, avoid frying; instead, bake, steam, or broil. Remove the skin from poultry before you cook it, and trim all visible fat from meat both before and after cooking. Choose lean cuts of meat, and broil them on a rack so the fat can drip away from the meat during cooking.

As discussed, eat three to six smaller meals during the day instead of just one large meal; your body will be less prone to store fat. Try not to overeat at any one meal — work more for balance, and provide your body with a steady source of fuel. Eat most of your calories in the morning, when you'll burn them as energy; eat fewer at night, when your body will be at rest.

**Exercise**

For the purposes of weight and fat loss, nothing beats aerobic exercise! Brisk walking, jogging, bicycling, swimming, and rowing are all good aerobic exercises. Choose the ones you like the best — the best exercise is the one you enjoy, because that's the one you'll do.

I recommend cross-training if you are serious about losing weight. What does it involve? Simply stated, it involves designing a program that includes a number of different sports and exercises.

What's the benefit?

There are several. First, you can train your entire body more fully. For example, if you combine running and swimming, you'll exercise both your lower and upper body. Even combining running and bicycling reaps different benefits: running works mostly the calves and hamstrings, and involves joint impact to the feet, ankles, and knees; bicycling stresses the muscles of the buttocks and the front of the legs and is a non impact exercise. Together, the two work the entire leg and ease some of the joint stress.

There are other benefits as well. For example, you won't overwork any one area of your body; as a result, you'll suffer fewer injuries. You'll have less tendency of getting bored with your exercise program. And, maybe most important, you won't burn out — instead of giving up and quitting, you will continue to make your exercise program work for you.

Almost any kind of exercise is beneficial. But if you want your exercise to help burn off pounds and fat, you need to follow some specific guidelines regarding frequency, duration, and intensity of exercise.

**Frequency.** If you want to lose weight, you need to exercise at least three to four times a week, even if you are just beginning an exercise program. Once you have adapted to your program or if you are an athlete who is already working out, you should try to exercise five to six times a week.

**Duration.** At a minimum your exercise workout should be for twenty to thirty continuous minutes, even if you are just beginning. If you are advanced, your workout should last for up to an hour or more if you want to lose weight.

**Intensity.** For weight and fat loss, you need to exercise continuously at 65 to 80 percent of your maximum heart rate, or within your "target zone." I explained in the first section how to calculate your target zone. If you want to lose body fat it is better to exercise for a longer period of time at the lower end of your target zone; in other words, you should exercise for an hour at 65 percent of your maximum heart rate rather than for half an hour at 80 percent of your maximum rate.

Intensity of exercise is one case in which less is better. Avoid the temptation to exercise at your maximum heart rate — you'll risk serious injury. The only people who should *occasionally* go toward 100 percent of maximum heart rate are competitive athletes, who may work this hard during race conditions — and who need to prepare for it. Even then, they should go all out no more than once a week.

Remember, as your fitness improves, you'll need to work harder to get your body to its target zone. That doesn't mean you should exercise at a higher heart rate — it just means that you'll need to expend more effort to reach the same heart rate. For example, a beginner who runs one mile in ten minutes will achieve a heart rate of 140 beats per minute. After she's been running for six months, she'll probably need to run the mile in eight minutes in order to achieve 140 beats per minute. And once she's been running regularly for two years, she'll need to run the mile in six minutes in order to get her heart rate to 140.

For best results, work at increasing your fitness level gradually; a good goal is to add no more than 5 percent per week in volume. That kind of gradual increase will help you avoid injury and soreness. Be patient — slow and steady wins this race every time! And remember: if you're older than thirty-five and have not ever exercised strenuously, get a physician's go-ahead before you start your exercise program. Why? There are certain heart beat irregularities that sometimes show up only during the elevated heart rates during exercise.

How much weight can you safely lose?

As discussed, a slow, gradual weight loss is the only safe way to trim your body fat. Experts agree that you should lose no more than one to two pounds per week if you hope to avoid illness and maintain your weight loss — and lose fat, not muscle.

### How to Gain Weight

Want to gain weight?

*Then don't use steroids.*

I can't stress the danger of steroids enough. There's a good reason why they are illegal drugs. There are a whole host of reasons why you should steer completely clear of steroids: among others, they have been shown to cause cancer, liver failure, kidney disease, high blood pressure, and heart irregularities. You might temporarily bulk up, but you're risking your life to do it — and nothing is worth the price of your good health and your precious life.

Plain and simple, say "no" to steroids.

Then how can an athlete gain the weight and muscle mass?

Slowly, for one thing. A safe weight *loss* is one to two pounds per week. The same rule of thumb applies for a weight *gain*. If you put on more than two pounds a week, you're gaining body fat — not muscle mass.

The first way to begin gaining muscle mass is to add calories to your diet; adding 500 to 1,000 per day is a good amount to aim for. Most of your additional calories should come from carbohydrates — fruits, vegetables, whole-grain cereals, breads, pasta, rice, potatoes, and so on. If you're trying to gain weight and muscle definition, you can step up your protein intake slightly: aim for about 20 to 25 percent of your total calories in *lean* protein (fish, poultry without skin, egg whites, and skim dairy products). *Whatever you do, avoid the temptation to beef up on fats.* Yes, they add calories — but they won't add muscle mass.

They'll just add body fat (and all sorts of other goodies, like an elevated cholesterol level and an increased risk of heart disease).

There are supplements on the market aimed at body builders and others who want to add muscle mass without adding body fat. Most are protein powders. If you decide to use one, you need to follow some guidelines.

First of all, read the label carefully. Some of the protein powders on the market are extremely high in fats (up to 15 grams per serving), high in simple sugars, and feature cheap animal byproducts as the source of protein. Avoid all three.

Second, make sure you use the protein powder according to label directions. It should never replace your meals, and should be used only as part of a healthy and balanced diet that is rich in carbohydrates, low in fat, and moderate in lean proteins.

Finally, this is another case where less is more. Avoid the temptation to figure that if *some* will build a little muscle mass, then a *whole bunch* will do the trick overnight. It won't. What it *will* do is overload your body with protein — and I've already talked about the dangers of that. An overload of protein is unhealthy and unwise, even for a growing body builder. Follow label directions as far as dosages go, and don't try to speed up the process.

Amino acids are the building blocks of protein — and of the twenty-two you need, you have to supply nine of them through diet. Your body can't manufacture them on its own. Amino acids contain the full spectrum of amino acids, so your body can choose the ones it needs to build and grow. That's a much safer, more reasonable approach than taking individual amino acids — as an example, L-tryptophan as an individual product was just removed from the market because it can cause blood disorders when taken alone.

### A Word About Injury ...

As an athlete, you're prone to injury — whether you're competing in your sport, working out to lose weight, trying to define muscle, or working to add muscle mass. You depend on your body being sound and strong, and it's frustrating to be cut down by any kind of injury.

What can you do?

Unfortunately, not much. The key with any kind of injury is *patience*. Rely on the advice of your physician or sports physiologist, and don't try to push too hard. You can't speed healing. What you can do is keep a positive attitude, resume mild exercise as your physician allows, and make sure you are eating a good balance of nutritious food. This is one time when you can slightly increase your protein, since it is essential to the healing process.

In a word, if you can't run, walk. If you can't walk, swim. You should not completely abandon your exercise and fitness program — you should simply find an exercise that will protect the injured limb from overuse and further injury. Your physician can give you some good guidelines; follow them.

Don't push yourself, but avoid the temptation to baby yourself. Be encouraged by small improvements, and remember that recovery is an active, not a passive, process. Experiment with ice, heat, massage, stretching, and maybe even anti-inflammatory medications. Work with your doctor or therapist for a speedy recovery.

Muscle sprains are a common injury for athletes, and it's essential that you understand how to treat them. Why? Because what you do in the first half hour after a sprain can affect the entire course of recovery.

The formula is a simple one: RICE. Rest. Ice. Compression. Elevation. As soon as possible after the injury occurs, pack it with ice; keep the ice pack on the injured area for twenty to thirty minutes. The ice will help reduce swelling (which can impair healing) and will relieve pain. *Never put ice directly on bare skin*; avoid frostbite injury by wrapping the ice in a towel or other protective wrapping.

Use the ice pack for twenty to thirty minutes at a time, with an hour or so between ice pack applications. After the first twenty-four to forty-eight hours, use heat on the sprain to stimulate the flow of blood to the area (increased blood flow will enhance healing).

If the sprain has occurred in an extremity, such as the ankle or wrist, elevate it to prevent swelling. If the sprain is serious, see your physician or sports physiologist so the area can be properly wrapped to avoid further injury.

I'll talk more about specific injuries in the physical fitness section!

# Physical Fitness and Training Principles

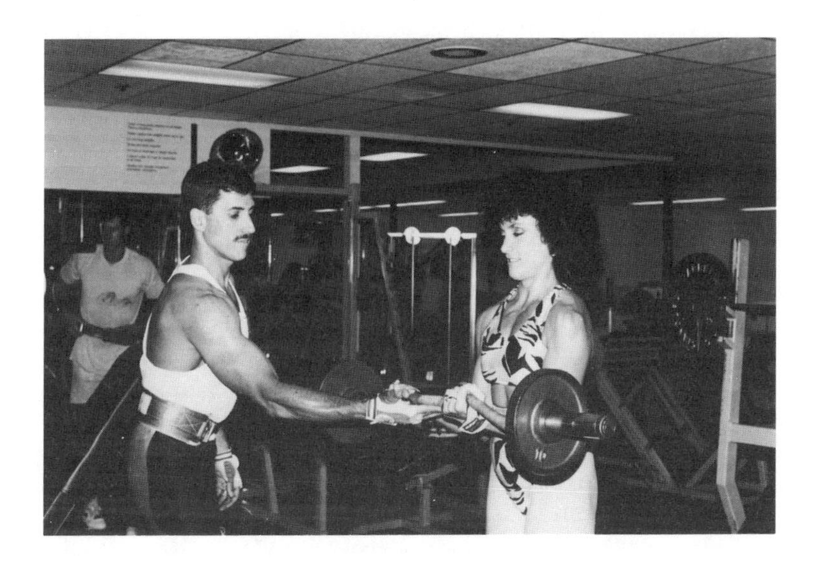

Okay — time to do your homework!

Why?

Before you begin any physical fitness or training program, you need to answer a basic question.

*Exactly what are your fitness goals?*

If you don't know now, you'd better find out. Why? Because the type of program you design and the intensity with which you work at it will depend on what your goals are. A forty-year-old who wants to lose extra weight and stay trim will approach the situation completely differently than a twenty-five-year-old who wants to complete in triathlons.

Take some time to figure out where you want to be a year from now. What do you want to be doing that is different from today's activities? How do you want to look — is it different than you look now? Is your main goal to lose weight? Bulk up muscles? Have more energy and endurance? Or to excel at a particular sport?

If you're exercising to lose weight, you'll want to stay in the lower end of your target zone — and you'll need to plan on spending more time. If you want to train as a competitive athlete, you'll need to train more often in the upper range of your target zone, and you'll need to be able to maintain a high workload.

Regardless of your fitness goals, there are some general principles that apply across the board. Following these principles will increase the effectiveness of your physical fitness program, no matter what your goal.

Above all, make sure you get a complete workout. How? There are four components of physical fitness: cardiovascular exercise (sometimes called "aerobic" exercise), muscular strength exercise, muscular endurance exercise, and flexibility (or "stretching") exercise. To get the full benefit of physical fitness, you need to incorporate all four into your fitness program.

Sound complicated?

It's not! In fact, all four can be easily incorporated into a thirty-minute workout session. Want an example? Stretch for a few minutes before and after each workout as part of your warm-up and cool-down routines; you'll incorporate flexibility exercise. Accomplish cardiovascular exercise by doing any large-muscle, continuous exercise for at least twenty minutes; brisk walking, jogging, bicycling, and swimming are all good examples. Bring in muscular strength and endurance exercises by using free weights, weight machines, or free calisthenic exercises (such as pushups, chinups, parallel bar dips, sit-ups, or leg lifts).

There you have it!

If you're a beginner, you might want to alternate your routines: do cardiovascular exercise one day, muscle strength/endurance exercises the next. Of course, you'll do flexibility exercises in the form of stretching each time you work out. As you become more fit, you can combine all four elements into a single workout. Just remember that everyone — including advanced athletes — needs to rest one day a week.

Remember, too, if you're thirty-five and just beginning a physical fitness program, check with your physician. You should have a stress electrocardiogram. Why? Because an estimated 85 percent of heart irregularities will not be detected on a resting EKG!

Before I discuss each specific type of exercise, I'd like to briefly go over some general training principles. These apply to any kind of exercise program, and can help you avoid injury and burnout.

First, follow the overload principle: give your body a challenge! Your body will only adapt and become stronger if you work it against loads greater than it normally encounters

Second, make your program specific. Your physical fitness program will be different than mine, because your goals are probably different than mine. Your program should be specific in carrying out your objectives — design a program that will strengthen the areas of your body you want to work with. Simply stated, tailor your program to meet your needs.

Third, vary your training. Don't choose just one activity (jogging, for example, or lifting weights). Do cross-training: select a number of different and complimentary activities. Why? To avoid boredom, for one thing. But there's an even more important reason: cross-training helps prevent overuse of any one body part, and will help you avoid injury.

Fourth, ease into your program. Start out slowly to avoid injury, soreness, and fatigue. Then gradually build up; I advocate adding no more than 5 to 10 percent to your fitness program each week.

Fifth, don't expect results overnight. Take a second look — and a skeptical one, at that — at anyone or any product that promises immediate results. Remember how long it took you to get out of shape: if you haven't exercised for months or years, you're not going to achieve your goals in a week or two. In general, it takes about four weeks of a conscientious, regular program before you will see any real fitness gain. Don't get discouraged — stick with it, and the rewards will come!

Sixth, never completely extend yourself. It's a mistake to "test" yourself to the limits. Why? Every time you do, you risk serious injury — and your recovery time is greater, too. Stick with the program you have outlined for yourself; training effects are cumulative, and will pay off as you gradually work toward your goal.

Finally, guard against overtraining. Monitor your pulse rate. Stay within your target zone! Keep an eye on your resting heart rate, too: an increase of 10 beats per minute in a resting pulse means that you are overtraining. Cut back. Rest at least one day a week, even if you have designed a very aggressive program. If you are going to compete, rest before your event — you should reduce your exercise for a racquetball match, a week for a marathon. Remember that training to the bitter end will deplete your body without giving you a better performance. And, above all, realize that *chronic pain and fatigue are signs that you need to slow down.* Pushing it will only result in injury.

**Cardiovascular Exercise**

Of the four components of physical fitness, cardiovascular exercise is the most important.

Why?

Cardiovascular exercise — a workout that increases your heart and lung capacity — brings with it all kinds of health benefits that you can't get with other activities. The result is not only a more physically fit body, but significantly increased health and longevity.

What are the benefits?

For one, you increase your body's ability to take up oxygen. That's a benefit both for workouts and for everyday living. Each task you do — climbing a flight of stairs, scrubbing a kitchen floor, running to catch a bus — feels easier. Overall, you have a greater supply of energy.

Cardiovascular exercise also slows down your resting heart rate (an effect called "bradycardia"). Why is that so important? Simple: your heart doesn't have to work as hard or beat as often to do the same amount of work.

Another benefit of cardiovascular exercise is that it helps control weight. Cardiovascular exercise is more efficient and burns more calories per minute than any other kind of exercise. There's an added benefit: cardiovascular exercise raises your metabolism. That's not all — it stays elevated after you stop exercising, which means you'll continue to burn calories after you exercise.

Cardiovascular exercise is good for your cardiovascular system: it helps develop a larger, stronger heart. It actually increases the chamber size of your heart and leads to the development of a larger capillary network. The end result? Your risk of heart disease is sharply reduced. You have an increased stroke volume, which means that your heart works more efficiently to pump more blood with each beat.

Still another benefit is that cardiovascular exercise can actually cause your body to manufacture a greater volume of blood. That means you'll have more red blood cells. And that means that your blood will carry more oxygen to the tissues of your body, resulting in better health and vitality.

Cardiovascular exercise can also actually alter your blood chemistry to prevent atherosclerosis, or the buildup of plaque and fat in the arteries. It lowers cholesterol levels, lowers the amount of low-density lipoproteins in the blood, and boosts the concentration of high-density lipoproteins (the "good" blood fats that help rid your body of cholesterol). When combined with a low-fat diet, cardiovascular exercise is the best cholesterol-buster around.

That's not the only benefit to the cardiovascular system: aerobic exercise also lowers blood pressure in people with hypertension. Many who have been on regular medication for high blood pressure find that exercise reduces or eliminates their need for drug therapy.

One of the greatest benefits of cardiovascular disease involves the muscles: they become much more capable of efficiently using oxygen. What does that mean to you? They are better at getting rid of lactic acid and wastes — and you experience much less muscle fatigue and soreness.

What is the best kind of cardiovascular exercise?

There is no "best" cardiovascular exercise. As I stated earlier, the best one is the one you like — because it's the one you will do. Brisk walking, jogging, bicycling, and swimming are good examples of cardiovascular exercise. You can also achieve excellent, effective cardiovascular exercise on a stationary bike, treadmill, or rowing machine. The key is that you need to choose an exercise that involves the large muscles of the body (the legs, back, shoulders, chest, and arms, for example) and that enables you to bring your heart rate to your target zone for at least *twenty continuous minutes*. Tennis uses the muscles of your whole body, for example, but it's not really an aerobic exercise. Why? Because the effort comes in spurts and is not continuous. My personal favorite exercise machine is the cross country ski simulator made by Nordic Track. It works upper and lower body at the same time in a smooth, non-impact fashion.

Stationary bikes, treadmills, and rowing machines can all

provide a great cardiovascular workout. The key is to invest in a quality machine and the *use it.* Use the machine to figure out what it takes to get your pulse to your target zone, and then determine how much effort you need to sustain to keep your heart working at that rate for at least twenty minutes. When you work indoors on machines, make sure you keep a water bottle nearby to guard against dehydration; use a fan, if needed, to keep yourself cooled off. And make sure to include a warm-up and cool-down set of stretching exercises, just as you would in any outdoor exercise.

Remember that calisthenics do *not* qualify as aerobic exercise. They simply don't use enough muscle mass or elevate the heart rate and metabolism sufficiently. Want a good example? I once did half a million sit-ups in fifteen weeks. That's 10,000 a day. At the end of the fifteen weeks, I did 52,003 sit-ups in just over thirty-two hours to set a new world record. And guess what? I was never fatter in my life. Even my abdominal muscles had very little definition. Why? I didn't change my eating habits; I was eating the same as I had when doing cardiovascular exercise. But my calisthenics didn't offer the benefits of aerobic exercise, and I paid the price.

What are the keys to good cardiovascular exercise? Let me briefly go over the basics:

**Type of exercise.** Choose any large-muscle, continuous aerobic exercise for cardiovascular fitness. The key is that your heart rate must stay elevated for at least twenty *continuous* minutes — no spurts of activity. Brisk walking, jogging, bicycling, swimming, aerobics, and cross-country skiing are all excellent choices. Just remember to keep your heart rate up for twenty continuous minutes; if you're bicycling, for example, try to choose level terrain so that you are pedaling at a constant rate instead of coasting down hills.

Remember the principle of cross-training. For the best results, choose a variety of cardiovascular exercises, and vary them; you'll reduce your risk of overuse and injury. Triathlons give us a good example of cross-training: you might want to combine jogging or running, bicycling, and swimming.

**Frequency.** To be effective, cardiovascular exercise must be performed at least three times a week — preferably more often. If you can, exercise on six days a week, and rest for one. Athletes and other professionals often train twice a day, six days a week.

**Duration.** To get the benefits of cardiovascular exercise, you need to do it for at least twenty continuous minutes; do it longer, if you can. If you're trying to lose weight, you should exercise at the lower end of your target zone, but you'll need to do it for about an hour. If you're a seasoned athlete, you might work out for several hours; bike racers and marathoners often exercise for two to five hours a day.

**Intensity.** As discussed, you need to exercise for at least twenty continuous minutes at 65 to 80 percent of your maximum heart rate (your "target zone"). To learn how to calculate your target zone, see my formula in the section on nutrition and health. It's important to measure your heart rate frequently during exercise so you can make sure your intensity is within range; count your pulse for ten seconds, then multiply by six to get your per-minute rate. A better method is using a heart rate monitor while you exercise.

Remember that younger people will need to work harder to achieve their target zone; older people can take it a little easier and still achieve their goal. Seasoned athletes can boost their target zone a little, training at about 80 to 85 percent of their maximum heart rate.

Remember, too, that it's important to warm up and cool down when you exercise.

In addition to stretching your muscles, you need to allow your heart five minutes to get up to speed and five minutes to gradually slow back down to a resting pulse after your workout. That means you'll need a total of thirty minutes to work out: twenty minutes in your target zone, and ten minutes total for warm-up and cool-down.

**Diet.** For full cardiovascular exercise benefits, accompany your workout with a diet that will also be heart-healthy. I've already discussed specific nutrition guidelines. For the optimum in heart health, remember to lower your total fat intake, increase the amount of polyunsaturated fats, increase the amount of fiber in your diet, lower the amount of cholesterol-containing foods you eat, lower your salt intake, and drink plenty of water.

**Warning signals.** Cardiovascular exercise, when done properly, is a fairly vigorous workout for your heart and lungs. *If at any time during aerobic exercise you feel dizziness, shortness of* *breath, or nausea, immediately stop exercising.* It's a sign you're overworking your cardiovascular system. If this happens more than once, you should check with your doctor before resuming your exercise program. If you have diabetes or hypoglycemia, make sure you eat before your workout. If you are diabetic, check with your doctor for advice on how to monitor insulin requirements as you work out.

**Strength Exercise**

While cardiovascular exercise provides the greatest health benefits, there are still some very good reasons to include strength training (sometimes called weight-lifting) in your exercise routine.

One good reason is physical appearance. Besides your skin, bones, and organs, your body has two basic components: muscle and fat. Strength exercise helps increase the amount of muscle for a firm, toned, attractive physical appearance. If you're a woman, don't worry about getting bulky muscles — use lighter weights with higher repetitions (at least fifteen per set) to increase muscle strength without increasing muscle bulk. Bulk requires not only very hard work, but fairly high levels of the male hormone testosterone — and very few women have enough testosterone to create bulk.

Another reason for strength training is to increase your capacity for physical activity. When you strengthen your muscles, you enable them to do things they couldn't do before — and to do them with greater ease.

Strength exercises also help increase your metabolic functioning. While they are not a key to rapid weight loss, strength exercises do improve the way your body utilizes calories. The improved metabolic effect doesn't stop when you put down the weights, either — it usually continues for a period after you have stopped exercising. Muscle is an active tissue that needs calories even at rest. Fat is inert and needs no energy to support it. More muscle burns more calories!

Strength exercises also help protect you against injury. How? When muscles are weak, they are more susceptible to injury; when they are tight and strong, they resist injury. Cardiovascular exercise also carries with it the risk of "muscle imbalance" — in other words, you may strengthen one group of muscles, but not the corresponding group. The common results can include lower back pain, runner's knee, swimmer's shoulder, shinsplints, stress fractures, and joint pain. If your strength exercises work all major muscle groups, you can avoid muscle imbalance and reduce your risk of injury.

Finally, strength exercises boost your athletic power. That's not limited to helping you toss a football farther or smack a racquetball harder — strength exercises will also give you the power you need to perform cardiovascular exercise. Think about it: all kinds of cardiovascular exercise require power (the power to run, to swim, to pedal a bicycle). The right kind of strength exercises can provide the power you need to improve your aerobic capacity without causing your muscles to become tight or sore.

You'll need to follow some general guidelines when doing strength exercises:

First, remember the principle of progressive overload. Start out with light weights until you perfect your technique, and then gradually move to heavier weights. Just remember to make the transition *gradually* so you will increase strength instead of risking injury. Keep revising your goals — always work toward crossing the next barrier!

Second, remember your warm-up. Warm-up is critical in strength exercises to prepare your muscles for the workout. If you fail to warm up, you risk muscle injury. Your warm-up should consist of gentle stretching of the muscle groups that you will be working; stretch the muscle just until you feel a good tension, and hold the stretch for up to thirty seconds *without bouncing*. Never jerk your muscles, and never stretch them until they are painful.

Third, use proper form at all times when working with weights or weight machines. If you can't lift the weight without sacrificing form, then the weight is too heavy; use a lighter weight until your muscles have strengthened. If you sacrifice form, you risk injury.

Fourth, don't work the same group of muscles on consecutive days; allow at least one to two days between workouts of muscle groups. For example, if you work your biceps on Monday, don't work them again until Wednesday or Thursday. Why? Strength exercises cause micro tears in the muscle. If you rest the muscle between workouts, get proper nutrition, and take appropriate supplements, your muscles will heal stronger than they were previously.

Fifth, train *intensely*. Except for your warm-up and cool-down exercises, every exercise should go to "failure" — in other words, until you can do no more repetitions. Sound hard? It is. Strength exercises require hard work, so be prepared when you go to the gym.

Should you work on free weights or weight machines?

Both give you a good workout, and each one has certain advantages if it is used properly. Free weights force you to use more supporting muscles for balance, give you a greater range of motion, and seem to enable the development of greater muscle mass. Machines offer greater safety, especially for people who are beginners or who exercise without a partner. Weight machines also offer a wide variety of exercises, and good-quality machines should be solidly built and move fluidly without binding. Choose whichever one works best for you in designing your strength exercise program.

What about letting a child lift weights? Generally, a child should not lift heavy weights until the age of sixteen or seventeen; prior to that age, the bone ends are still soft (to allow for complete growth), and damage can occur that will impair the growth process. Younger children should be encouraged to build a good aerobic base with cardiovascular exercise and sports like bicycling, soccer, basketball, swimming, and tennis. Children can tone muscles with calisthenics, such as sit-ups and push-ups, and can use light weights. How can you tell that a weight is light enough? A child should be able to perform at least fifteen repetitions if the weight is right.

To maximize your strength gains, lift heavy weights for fewer repetitions for the greatest benefit. The key is intensity — push yourself until you can't do another repetition. If the weights are too light, you'll do too many sets and too many exercises. The result is overtraining and low intensity.

A good strength program should follow these guidelines:

**Repetitions.** Try for six to eight repetitions per set; if you can't do that many, the weight is probably too heavy for you. Fewer repetitions will help you develop strength, but will not increase muscle size.

**Sets.** Set a goal of doing three to four sets for each exercise.

**Exercises.** You should try for a maximum of three to four exercises for each body part, and should aim for ten to twelve total exercises each session. This kind of a program will give you a good workout, and you'll have noticeable strength gains within a few weeks.

Vary your exercises so that each group of muscles gets a workout every two to three days. For the chest, use the flat bench, incline, decline, and pec deck. For arms, do bicep curls and tricep extensions. For shoulders, try military or overhead presses and flies. For the entire upper body, do bar dips, push-ups, and pull-ups. For abdominal muscles, do sit-ups, leg lifts, and crunches. And for the leg muscles, do leg press, squats, leg extensions and curls, and calf raises.

Full-range exercises are the most beneficial. Isometric exercises can be a good addition to your fitness program, however, because they require little time, a minimum of room, and no equipment. If you are training for athletic competition, try to keep your strength training exercises at a constant speed; move rapidly from one set to the next without letting your heart rate or intensity level drop. Isokinetic devices such as the Nordic Fitness chair are excellent for this purpose.

## Endurance Exercises

Muscle strength and muscle endurance are closely related: when one improves, the other one generally does, too. Generally, the difference between the two types of exercise is in repetition —when exercising to improve muscle endurance, you need to do as many repetitions as possible.

Muscular endurance is defined as the ability to perform an exercise for either many repetitions or for a long period of time. It differs from muscular strength (which is the ability to perform one maximal effort) and from cardiovascular endurance (which is endurance that is limited to the heart, lungs, and circulatory system). Muscular endurance exercise is demanding — your body needs to keep going for long periods, be as efficient as possible, not waste energy, and not accumulate waste fatigue products (such as lactic acid).

The best way to train for muscular endurance is with resistance exercises — and they can be free weights, weight machines, or calisthenics (such as pull-ups, sit-ups, or push-ups).

The goal of endurance exercise is to be able to perform increasingly more repetitions of the exercise. Except in unusual circumstances, speed is not important.

Because speed is not important, you should "ease into" the exercise. Your initial pace should be slow to allow your body to gradually adjust to the increased energy demands. If you begin exercising at too great a speed, your body will incur an oxygen debt and your muscles will begin to churn out lactic acid. When lactic acid builds up, you'll experience soreness and muscle fatigue — and the number of repetitions you can do will be severely curtailed.

Endurance exercises need to be performed for long periods of time; some athletes do endurance exercises for up to ten hours at a stretch or more. Your goal, again, is to do as many repetitions as you can. For a beginner, aim for two or three sets of exercise, fifteen or more repetitions of each, at least three times a week.

*Remember:* High weight and low repetitions boosts your strength; lower weight and higher repetitions boosts your endurance.

As with strength exercises, you should perform endurance exercises no more often than every other day — your muscles need time to recover and repair between exercise sessions.

What kinds of exercises are good for endurance?

A variety of free-weight exercises can be used. Try bench press and flies for the chest; curls and tricep extension for the arms; military press and flies for the shoulders; pullups, chins, and rowing for the back; and squats, dead lifts, and good mornings for the legs. Use light weights; you should be able to do twelve to twenty-five repetitions of each exercise. If you can't do at least twelve repetitions, your weight is too heavy for endurance exercise — move down to a lower weight.

Most types of calisthenics work well for endurance exercise; again, the key is to do as many repetitions as you can, not to exercise at a fast pace. One word of caution about sit-ups, a favorite endurance exercise: make sure you are doing your sit-ups properly to protect against lower back pain. Three factors add up to proper form when doing sit-ups: keep your knees bent, keep your chin to your chest, and keep your back rounded. Pretend you have a heavy weight on your stomach that is pressing your lower back into the floor; force the small of your back against the floor, and never allow your back to arch while you are doing sit-ups.

If you do injure your back, avoid straight leg raises, full sit-ups, and other exercises that stress the back and abdomen. Begin with some very slow and controlled crunches and bent-leg raises while hanging from a bar; slowly and gradually increase the repetitions and intensity as your back muscles and abdominal muscles strengthen.

A final note about endurance exercise: *if an exercise hurts, don't do it.* Pain is a sure signal from your body that you need to ease up.

**Flexibility Exercises**

Flexibility is defined as the range of motion that is possible around any given joint; flexibility exercises are those that help increase the range of motion. Flexibility tends to decrease with age; older people gradually get stiffer, and their muscles gradually get shorter and tighter.

Age isn't the only reason why flexibility exercises are needed, though. Athletes who overuse one part of their body lose flexibility; runners may get tight hamstrings, and weight lifters may get tight pectorals. The answer is flexibility exercises — gentle stretching exercises that return range of motion to normal.

Every exercise program should include at least ten minutes of flexibility exercises — five minutes during the warm-up period, and five minutes during the cool-down period. These flexibility exercises not only help restore range of motion, but prevent muscle injury and cramping.

Stretching exercises are "joint specific" — in other words, you need to individually stretch the muscles around each separate joint. Obviously, you can't stretch the muscles around every joint in your body in a mere five-minute warm-up period. Which ones do you choose? It depends on the activity you're about to do. Stretch the muscles you will be using in your exercise, and stretch the muscles around the joints that will get the most impact during your workout. If you will be running or bicycling, stretch your quads, hamstrings, calves, and lower back. If you will be swimming or playing racquetball, stretch the muscles of your arms, shoulders, and chest. If you will be lifting weights, stretch the muscles you will be working on during that session.

Simply stated, stretching is often the most important — but the most overlooked — part of an exercise program. Stretching for five minutes before your workout helps prevent muscle injury — pre-stretched muscles are longer, more limber, stronger, and faster than muscles that have not been stretched. Five minutes of stretching after your workout prevents your muscles from tightening up, reduces soreness, speeds recovery time, and helps flush out waste products (such as lactic acid).

How should you stretch?

Stretching exercises should be slow and steady — and they should be static, which means they should be done without bobbing, bouncing, or jerking. Bouncing and jerking actually activate the muscle spindles, which results in greater muscle contraction. What happens then? Your muscles actually get shorter instead of longer — and you've defeated the purpose of flexibility exercise.

The stretch should be felt in your muscle, not at the joint. If you can feel the stretch at the joint, you are overstretching: you will pull the non-elastic ligaments at the joint. These don't return to their original length, so you run the risk of making your joints unstable. The obvious end result could be joint injury.

Each stretch should be gently done until you feel a good stretch, but not until you feel pain. Proper flexibility exercises should never be painful! When you reach the proper degree of stretch, hold it for at least thirty seconds *without any movement.* You should feel a gentle pull. Release the stretch after at least thirty seconds, and move to the next muscle that needs to be stretched.

When you first begin flexibility exercises, you might feel discouraged because of tightness; you might not be able to stretch your muscles very far. As with all exercise, be patient. If you continue to do regular flexibility exercises, you should notice significant improvement as your body begins to adapt. If you faithfully do stretches before and after each workout, you should begin to see results in three to four weeks.

**Special Exercise Considerations**

The exercise guidelines I've outlined in this section are for average, healthy people of all skill levels. They apply to beginners as well as to advanced athletes — duration and intensity obviously increase as an athlete gains experience and becomes more fit.

There are some special considerations, however, in recommending an exercise program for a pregnant woman or for the elderly.

**Exercise During Pregnancy**

Regardless of what your situation is, *consult your physician before beginning any exercise program if you are pregnant.* If you have been exercising before pregnancy, your physician will probably give you the go-ahead to continue your usual or a slightly modified exercise program. If you have not been exercising prior to pregnancy, your physician will need to determine whether you can safely start and how much exercise you should attempt.

Barring complications, you can probably do stretching exercises, toning exercises, and cardiovascular exercises through most of your pregnancy. Swimming, bicycling, and walking are good aerobic exercises that can be safely done by most pregnant women. Jogging, running, and other high-impact exercises (such as jumping jacks) may not be appropriate; your physician can best advise you.

Even if you are given a green light for cardiovascular exercises during pregnancy, you need to stay aware of your body and the changes that are taking place. Stay in the lowest end of your target range to prevent depriving your growing baby of oxygen. As your pregnancy advances, you'll be able to work less and less to reach your target range. Never do any exercise that leaves you breathless, that causes pain, or that makes you uncomfortable. *Stop exercising immediately if you feel dizzy, winded, or nauseated.*

Check with your physician during the last stages of your pregnancy. You will probably need to slow down, and you may even need to curtail or stop your exercise program until after your baby is born. Never allow yourself to become dehydrated; drink plenty of fluids before, during, and after workouts.

**Exercise for Older People**

High-impact exercises, such as running, jogging, and most aerobic dance, are often painful and difficult for older people to do. But that doesn't mean they should stop exercising! There are plenty of fun and beneficial low-impact exercises that will provide fitness without causing pain.

Exercise is particularly important for the elderly. Why? Strength exercises prevent the muscles from shrinking and can even reverse some muscle atrophy. As we age, we tend to lose flexibility — and stretching exercises help to preserve range of motion and prevent joint stiffness. Exercise is especially important to elderly women, since it can help slow calcium loss from the bone and can in many cases slow or prevent osteoporosis.

As age increases, it take less effort to reach the exercise target zone. If you are older, pay special attention to your heart rate during exercise. Keep it at the low end of your target zone, and never exercise so hard that you can't carry on a comfortable conversation while you are exercising. Slow down if you start to feel breathless or winded.

Aerobic exercises especially suited to older people include walking, swimming, bicycling, and cross-country skiing. Low-impact aerobic classes are also offered in many areas; these kinds of aerobic exercises will not cause joint pain. Older people can also do weight training; ask the counselor at the gym or health club to help you develop a routine that is appropriate to your age and physical abilities.

### Common Injury Problems

Exercise causes you to work a little harder than you have before — and, by its very nature, it can leave you susceptible to injury. You can guard against injury and substantially reduce your risk by following the guidelines I've given in these sections.

When injury does occur, give yourself time to recover fully before going back to your full fitness routine. Injured joints and muscles need rest — and you can't speed the healing process. You can safely take care of minor injuries, but make sure to consult a physician for any major illness or injury.

In my experience, I've seen three very common injuries among three different kinds of athletes: shinsplints among runners, lower back pain among cyclists, and swimmer's shoulder among swimmers. All three can be safely treated by following these guidelines:

**Shinsplints.** If you suffer from shinsplints, stop running or jogging until the pain goes away. You can continue your fitness program, but swim or cycle instead. Once the pain subsides, you can start running again. Cut your mileage down, and run on soft surfaces, such as grass. Wear well-cushioned shoes that provide plenty of support, and ease up your pace so you don't run hard downhill.

To prevent shinsplints from occurring, make sure you stretch the muscles in your calves well both before and after running. Use strength or endurance exercises to develop all the muscles around your calves equally — shinsplints are caused by a muscle imbalance in the lower leg; the calf muscles being stronger and tighter than those of the shin.

To relieve the pain from shinsplints, rub ice on your shins for fifteen to thirty minutes at a time. Take buffered aspirin to relieve pain. Doing gentle stretching exercises for your lower legs can also help relieve the pain of shinsplints.

**Cyclist's lower back pain.** Lower back pain or tightness in a cyclist can be caused by improper bicycle adjustment, failure to do adequate stretching exercises, and fatigue.

If your seat or handlebars are not adjusted properly for your body, you can start feeling pain in your lower back. Take your bike to a shop and have an expert evaluate the seat and handlebar position in relationship to your body. Also let the expert know what kind of terrain you ride on and how long your workouts are. He or she can make the proper adjustments to your bicycle; often that alone will solve the problem.

A cyclist who fails to do proper stretching exercises can also get pain or tightness in the lower back. Make sure that you spend a full five minutes (or more) doing gentle stretches before you begin to cycle; concentrate on the muscles in your calves, thighs, and lower back. Be sure to keep your abdominal muscles strong to avoid muscle imbalances.

Lower back pain can also be the result of fatigue. Change your hand position on the handlebars frequently, and ride in and out of the saddle to prevent fatigue. If you feel like your lower back is beginning to tire, stretch while riding by standing with your legs straights and your upper body leaning over the handlebars.

Finally, give your body a chance to adapt to bicycling. Build up your time and mileage gradually. Cycling should be fun, not painful!

**Swimmer's shoulder.** Swimmer's shoulder is a common

condition among people who swim for exercise, and is usually due to overuse of the shoulder muscles. As a result, the small muscles and tendons of the shoulder get irritated, and pain occurs.

To treat swimmer's shoulder, avoid any movement that is painful; switch to different strokes or limit your swimming to kicking movements. If you can't find a stroke that is not painful, try some other form of exercise until your shoulder feels better.

Put ice packs on your painful shoulder for twenty to thirty minutes at a time, once or twice a day, to relieve inflammation. You can also take buffered aspirin, which will help relieve the pain and which will also reduce the inflammation. As the injured shoulder starts to feel better, begin a series of gentle stretching exercises to help restore flexibility and stretch the muscle. Remember — never stretch until it hurts!

When you begin swimming again, take a little extra time for warm-up and cool-down stretching exercises, especially those in your shoulder and back. Start out at a gradual pace, and allow your body to readapt to the movements of swimming before you reach full pace again.

**Exercise Burnout**

No discussion on exercise would be complete without a few words about burnout — the point at which you overtrain and, consequently, lose interest.

How can you determine whether you are exercising too much — and, therefore, are a candidate for burnout?

Unfortunately, there's no set formula to determine how much exercise is right for any one person. Each of us is an individual, and each body reacts differently to the various stresses that are a part of physical exercise. There *are* some questions you can ask yourself that might help you determine for yourself whether you are overdoing it:

Are you overtired or feeling undue fatigue? Any fitness workout will temporarily leave you feeling a little tired, but you should quickly feel an increase in energy. Exercise done at the proper rate and intensity should leave you feeling refreshed, not worn out. Bone-weary fatigue is a sign that you're doing too much.

Are you catching more colds than usual? If so, you're wearing your body out and your resistance is low. What about injuries? If you are suffering a series of nagging injuries, you probably need to cut back.

Do you look forward to your workouts with enthusiasm — or do you dread them? Your own emotions are a good key to how you're doing.

Finally, how is your performance? Have you noticed a gradual improvement, or are you staying about the same? Worse, are you backsliding? Exercise that is good for you will bring about improvement; if you don't notice even slight improvement, something's wrong.

So what can you do?

First of all, cut back on the amount you are exercising. Get more rest. Make sure you're getting plenty of sleep at night, and watch what you eat. Good nutrition and adequate rest can go far in helping against burnout.

If you've been exercising five or six days a week, cut down to three or four. Take a day off between each exercise session for awhile until you feel completely rested.

Monitor your resting pulse rate. Before you get out of bed in the morning, lie completely still for two or three minutes. Then take your pulse, and record it. Take your resting pulse rate each morning, and learn what is normal for you. One sure sign of overtraining or too much exercise is an increase in your resting pulse rate. If your resting pulse rate goes up by as much as ten beats per minute, cut back on your exercise and get more rest.

When you are exercising properly, you should show improvement. You may not always improve each time you exercise, but you should have an overall pattern of improvement. If you're not improving, you're probably too tired. Avoid the temptation to exercise even harder or faster in an attempt to make up for lost time. Instead, take a break for a few days, and start out again at a slower pace.

Above all, *enjoy yourself!* Exercise should be fun — something you look forward to and enjoy doing. Design a fitness program that delights your senses. Choose activities you enjoy, and experience the joy that comes from a well-tuned, fit body!

The Fitness Formula adds up to a balanced fitness program — one that incorporates strength, flexibility, and aerobic conditioning as well as a sound nutritional base, enough rest and reduced stress levels and bad habits. Incorporate this formula into your life and experience the joy of the fitness lifestyle. This is not a one week or one month program, but one for the rest of your life.

For more information on personal training and other related fitness products, phone (408) 578-1302 or write to:

P.O. Box 23312
San Jose, CA 95153

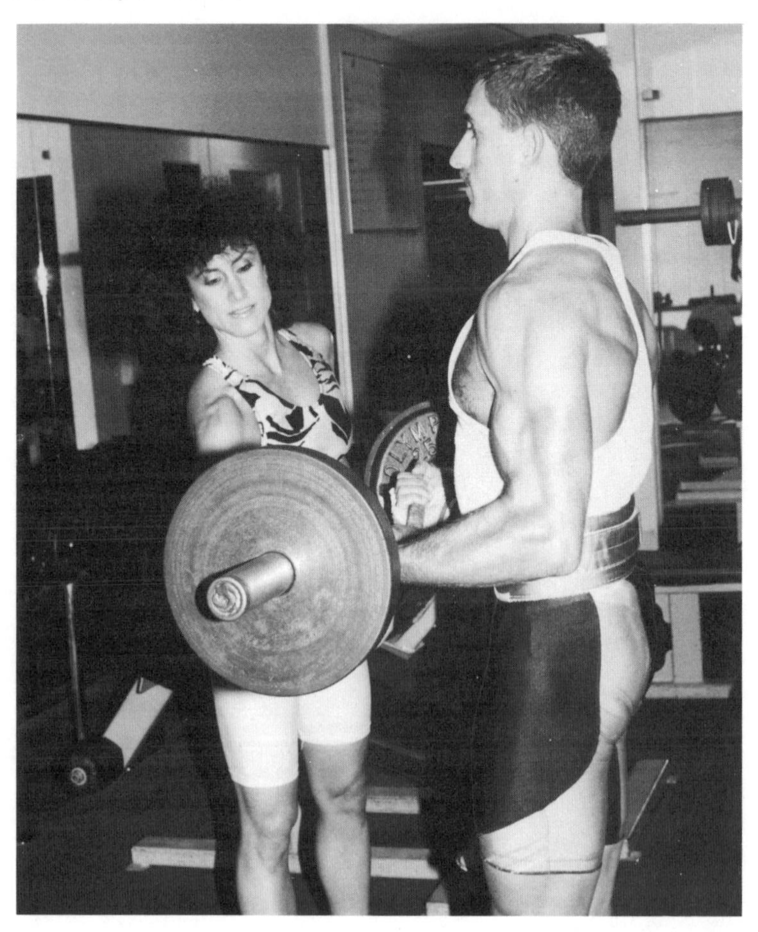

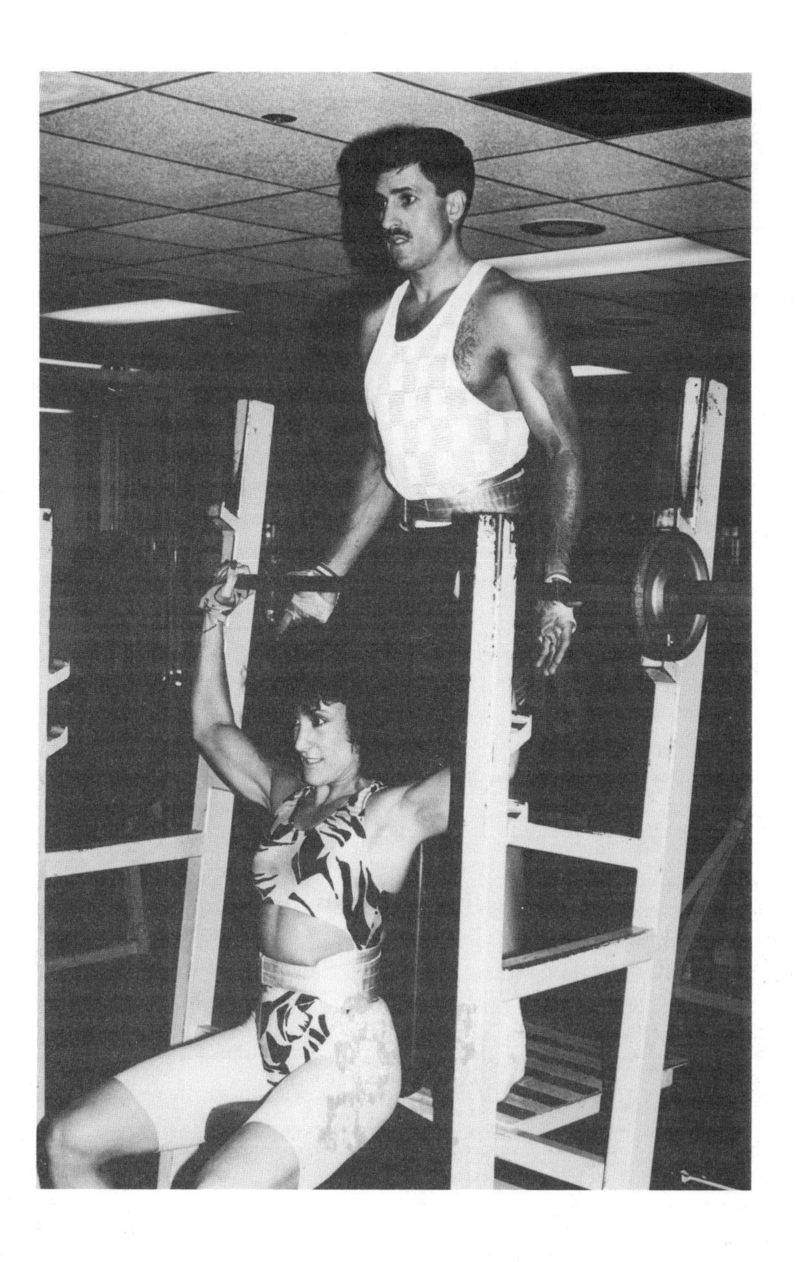